P9-BYO-455

Marla Heller, MS, RD

The DASH Diet
Action Plan

Amidon Press
Northbrook, Illinois

The DASH Diet Action Plan

All rights reserved.

Copyright @ 2005 by Marla Heller, MS, RD

The nutrition advice in this book is based on the DASH diet,
developed in the National Institutes of Health studies. It is not
intended to replace advice or treatment provided by your
physician. Please consult with your physician before making
any dietary changes. The author disclaims any liability arising
directly or indirectly from The DASH Diet Action Plan.

Nurtritional analyses on the menus in this book were obtained
from Nutritionist Pro, First DataBank.

Library of Congress Catalog Card Number: 2004117078

No part of this book may be reproduced or transmitted in any
form or by any means, electronic or mechanical, including
photocopying, recording, or by any information storage, and
retrieval system, without express written consent from the
publisher. For information, contact: Amidon Press, 520 Lake-
Cook Rd, Ste 280, Deerfield, IL 60015.

ISBN 0-9763408-0-1

Published March, 2005
Deerfield, Illinois
Amidon Press

Printed in the United States of America
10 9 8 7 6 5 4 3 2 1

Table of Contents

Acknowledgments

Many people have helped and supported me in preparing this book. First, I received research support and ideas for menu plans from two dietetic interns from the University of Illinois at Chicago, Andrea Denk and Susan Nordmark. Heidi Hartman, a dietetic intern from the University of Delaware performed much of the work in developing the analyses of the menu plans.

Susan Moores provided editing support on early drafts of several chapters of the book.

I was introduced to the DASH Diet by Shiriki Kumanyika, PhD, RD, who has extensive research background in management of hypertension, and was involved in the initial development of the DASH Diet concept. Shiriki was also my master's thesis advisor.

I also had the pleasure of arranging for Marlene Most, PhD, RD, speak at an Illinois Dietetic Association meeting, to provide more details about the DASH Diet research. She was instrumental in the design of the DASH Diet, one of the lead researchers, and is published frequently on the DASH Diet research.

My clients continue to provide me with the opportunity to learn how better to support dietary behavior change and help people with fitting healthy eating into hectic lives.

I continue to be grateful for the superior education and continuing guidance I have received in this, my second career, from my professors at Dominican University (Judy Beto, PhD, RD, and

Betsy Holli, PhD, RD) and at the University of Illinois at Chicago (Bob Reynolds, PhD, Phyllis Bowen, PhD, RD, Savitri Kamath, PhD, RD).

I also greatly benefitted from my students in the introductory foods classes and the nutrition education and counseling classes. They help me with developing recipes, some of which are found in the book, and in designing programs that help people adopt sustainable behavior changes.

My graduate course work in health behavior change theory and measurement have also helped me sharpten my focus on helping people make sustainable behavior change, and using research methods to evaluate the outcome of using a book for promoting behavior change. My epidemiology course work has reinforced the importance of controlling the epidemics of hypertension, heart disease, type 2 diabetes, and obesity.

And finally, I want to thank my husband, Richard, who has supported me in my endeavors over the five years it took to complete the book. He has been a never ending source of encouragement, support, and love and I am truly grateful to him.

Chapter 1 Conquering Hypertension and Heart Disease – the DASH Diet Plan

When you were a child, your grandmother probably told you to drink your milk, eat your fruits and vegetables, and go outside and play. This is still great advice, and shows that our fundamental ideas of good nutrition hold up over time.

The DASH diet is a "new" healthy eating plan, that has been proven to help reduce blood pressure. It was developed in major research studies funded by the National Institutes of Health, as the "Dietary Approaches to Stop

> **What is a Diet?**
>
> A diet is not just a plan for losing weight, a diet refers to the way that we eat. Any eating pattern is a diet.

Hypertension" (DASH). It is a diet based on the same great advice that our grandmother's generation lived by, which somehow, today's Americans seem to have forgotten.

When you follow the DASH plan, you will eat lots of fruits and vegetables, along with low fat dairy foods, lean meat, poultry, and fish, nuts and beans, and whole grains. The plan is low in saturated fat and cholesterol, it has a moderate amount of protein, and is rich in vitamins, minerals and fiber.

In addition to lower blood pressure, a diet based on the DASH foods is associated with lower risk of heart disease, stroke, and cancer. The DASH diet can support reaching and maintaining a healthy weight. No conflicting information, no magic combinations, no forbidden foods – just fabulous healthy eating.

Understanding Blood Pressure

Over 50 million Americans have high blood pressure. It is the leading cause of heart attacks and strokes. If your blood pressure goes too low you may feel lightheaded. If it goes too high there might not be any symptoms, or it could trigger a stroke. If blood pressure remains high, it can lead to congestive heart failure, kidney failure, hardening of the arteries, stroke, and other complications.

You might not have learned that you had high blood pressure until your physician detected it in a routine physical exam. You probably had no symptoms. You may not be able to detect that your blood pressure is high unless you check it on a regular basis. Since you often don't feel that anything is wrong, you might not keep it as well controlled as your physician would like. This is one of the reasons that hypertension has been called the "silent killer."

Our blood pressure is composed of 2 numbers. Systolic is the "top" number and diastolic is the "bottom" number. If our blood pressure is "120 over 80," the 120 is the systolic pressure, and 80 is the diastolic.

Blood Pressure Definitions

Normal: Systolic 90-119 and diastolic 60-79.
Prehypertension: Systolic 120-139 and diastolic 80-89.
Stage I hypertension: Systolic 140-159 and/or diastolic 90-99.
Stage II hypertension: Systolic 160 or higher and/or diastolic 100 or greater.

Blood pressure is considered to be high (hypertension) if systolic is higher than 140, or if diastolic is more than 90. (Your physician might consider you to have high blood pressure at slightly lower numbers, if there are other medical complications to consider.) A new category of "prehypertension" has been identified as systolic blood pressure between 120-139, or diastolic 80 - 90. When blood pressure is high, it forces our heart to beat harder to move the blood against more pressure and can cause premature hardening or other damage to the arteries.

High blood pressure is not an equal opportunity disease. Men are at higher risk than women with the same blood pressure. Blacks and older people will also be at higher risk than non-blacks or younger people with the same blood pressure readings. This makes it even more important to control hypertension

Blood pressure can be high for unknown reasons, which is called essential hypertension. It can also be elevated due to another disease process such as overproduction of certain hormones or kidney disease. This is called secondary hypertension, since it occurs secondary to another disease.

Why DASH?

Research sponsored by the National Institutes of Health has shown that this healthy diet can lower blood pressure as much as medication. Results are quick, with many people seeing lower blood pressure in only 14 days with the DASH diet. Adding weight loss (when needed), exercise and other healthy lifestyle choices further improves the blood pressure benefits. Why does the DASH diet make such a difference? And how does it differ from the average American diet?

A diet that is rich in minerals, high in fiber and low in saturated fat can help lower blood pressure. Many of the beneficial nutrients are found in fruits and vegetables along with low-fat dairy foods, all of which are lacking in the typical American diet.

The food guide pyramid (developed by the USDA and the US Department of Health and Human Services) recommends having 2 - 4 fruits and 3 - 5 vegetables each day. The DASH diet recommends 4 - 5 fruit and 4 - 5 vegetable servings each day. This may seem especially daunting when you realize that only about half of us even have one serving of fruit or fruit juice each day. And frequent meals away from home make it difficult to include enough fruits and vegetables in our meals. Is the DASH plan something that we can incorporate in a real life, with many meals eaten in restaurants or fast food places, and with little time for exercise? This book will help you with creative ideas to boost the health quotient of your daily routine, even if you are always on the run.

The DASH plan will help you use healthy foods and other actions to aid in management of your blood pressure. Will it help you eliminate or reduce the need for medication? Only your doctor can evaluate that question. Will it help you become more healthy? That it can do. We know that people who follow a diet low in saturated fat, rich in fruits, vegetables, legumes and other plant protein foods have reduced risk of heart disease and cancer. Exercise, smoking cessation, and moderate consumption of alcohol (if you drink) can provide additional cardiovascular health benefits. So, you have much to gain from choosing to follow the DASH plan.

Why not just take a supplement? If we could just find out what the key components were, it seems that it would be much easier to just pop a pill. However, scientific studies attempting to use supplements to control blood pressure have mostly failed. There is something in the mix of nutrients and other food components that appear to be protective against many diseases. This will be covered in more detail in several of the chapters in this book, including the chapter discussing the effects of sodium and other minerals on blood pressure.

At the heart of this book is a model menu plan which will show you how to put the DASH diet into effect. It will give you concrete examples of how you can add more fruits and vegetables to your diet, even if many of your meals are eaten away from home or if you are a picky eater. The menu plan in this book is full of fabulous meals, and dashes the belief that everything that tastes great is bad for you. You will find ways to add many foods that you thought would not be allowed in a healthy diet. If a healthy eating plan doesn't include your favorites, chances are you will not be able to follow it for very long.

DASH and More

Weight loss is often a critical component of blood pressure control. The DASH diet makes it easy to lose weight, since many of the DASH diet foods are more filling than empty calorie foods that many people over consume. You will learn how to determine your healthy weight, and how to adapt the DASH diet to meet your calorie needs. The satisfying eating plans in this book will make it easier than you think to lose weight. Exercise is another challenge in our over scheduled lives. A commitment to your health can be sustained with the easy-to-follow tips presented in this book.

Eat Well, Feel Great, Be Healthy

The DASH plan is a way of eating and living that you will want to continue. It will give you more energy and help you avoid the negative feelings that come from overeating foods that are high in calories but aren't so rich in nutrients. Exercise will rid you of that sluggish feeling that goes with a "couch potato" lifestyle. You will find ways to customize the plan for your own personal tastes, to make it something that you can really live with.

Many people with high blood pressure have other medical conditions, including heart disease. Fortunately, the DASH plan will also benefit many of these other conditions. Since it is high in fiber and rich in vitamins and minerals, it can help lower cholesterol, may make it easier to control blood sugar, and may reduce the risk of certain types of cancer.

Many of the risk factors for heart disease can be changed by making diet and lifestyle changes. You can quit smoking, control blood pressure, lower your cholesterol, lose weight, and get more active. And diet may help reduce newly identified risk factors for heart disease such as homocysteine and

C-reactive protein (a marker of inflammation).

Take Action

Now is the time to open your mind about the possibility of improving your health, by choosing to include more fruits and vegetables, other healthy foods and exercise in your day. This isn't the traditional diet message that focuses on the "bad foods" which should be eliminated from your diet. This is a positive message about adding great healthy foods to give you a pay off in improved blood pressure control, and improved health.

Heart disease risk factors
Controllable
1. Cigarette smoking
2. Hypertension
3. High cholesterol
4. Low HDL (good cholesterol)
5. Obesity
6. Diabetes
7. Sedentary
Not controllable
1. Family history of early heart disease
2. Age 45+ for men, and 55+ for women
Additional risk factors
1. High homocysteine
2. High C-reactive protein

Buying this book was your first step. The chapters will provide you with many tools to reach your goals. Menu plans let you translate the DASH diet into action. Adding on exercise, weight control, and other lifestyle changes will maximize the benefits. For people who want to understand more about healthy foods, there are chapters highlighting healthy carbs, fats, and protein-rich foods. Chapters on other nutrients show how they help promote health. For the vegetable phobics, we will coax you into expanding your diet with new choices. A kitchen make-over will help set the stage for success. And there is a chapter to help you with making your new eating and exercise habits into a life-long commitment.

Get ready to enjoy healthy eating and a healthy lifestyle, while reaping the rewards in feeling great!

Chapter 1 DASHboard

1. Your grandmother told you to drink your milk, eat your fruits and vegetables, and go outside and play. It is still valuable nutrition advice.
2. Over 50 million Americans have high blood pressure, and another 45 million have "pre-hypertension."
3. Even moderately high blood pressure is linked to increased risk of stroke, heart disease, heart failure, and kidney failure.
4. A diet rich in fruits, vegetables, and low-fat dairy foods can help you lower your blood pressure in 14 days.
5. Exercise, smoking cessation, moderate alcohol consumption, and weight loss can support lowering blood pressure.

Tracking my Personal DASH Diet Action Plan:

Current   **Target**
Blood pressure: _____   _____
Cholesterol: _____   _____
LDL: _____   _____
HDL: _____   _____
Triglycerides: _____   _____

Chapter 2 Your Personal DASH Diet Design

A typical day's DASH menu at 2000 calories looks like a decadent feast. When you approach a new diet by focusing on the foods you include, rather than on exclusions, it becomes pleasurable and fun to follow. The following typical day shows you how this happens.

Breakfast
Freshly Squeezed Orange Juice
Wheaties® with Skim Milk Topped with Raspberries
Cinnamon Raisin English Muffin with a Smear of Light Cream Cheese

Lunch
Turkey and Light Swiss Cheese on Whole Wheat, Smothered with Cranberry Sauce, Topped with Romaine Lettuce Leaves
Minestrone Soup
Cole Slaw

Snack
Nectarine
Handful of Almonds

Dinner
Italian Bread Dipped in Olive Oil

Grilled Salmon with Barbecue Sauce
New Petite Red Potatoes
Haricots Verts Dusted with Crushed Hazelnuts
Hearts of Romaine Salad Spiked with Grape
Tomatoes, Olive Oil Vinaigrette
Very Berry Sundae
(Strawberries, Blueberries, and Blackberries on
Light Vanilla Frozen Yogurt)

What are the easy-to-make changes that boosted the DASH foods in this diet? Fruit was added to make a sweet topping for cereal, a refreshing afternoon snack, and a luscious dessert at dinnertime. Lunch packed in two vegetable servings with a vegetable-stuffed soup and crisp cole slaw. The dinner plate includes potatoes, the very thin French green beans known as *haricots verts*, and a green and red salad. Light dairy foods show up at breakfast, on the lunchtime sandwich, and to make a satisfying sundae for dessert at dinner. Unexpected "real food" toppings include regular salad dressing at dinner, olive oil for the Italian bread, mayonnaise on the cole slaw, tangy cranberry sauce to spice up the all too familiar turkey sandwich, a handful of almonds for a snack, and crushed hazelnuts sprinkled on the green beans.

In this section we will show you how to make the DASH diet work for you. You will see how many servings add up to the right calories for your needs.

You will get specific tips to make the process more intuitive. Complementing this overview are 28 days of menu plans in Chapter 3, tips for staying on track while including restaurant meals in chapter 4, and weight loss support in chapter 5. Whether you want to cook most of your meals or eat away from home, you can DASH with ease.

This book will help make following the DASH diet as simple as adding key foods, choosing light and lean, and managing portions.

Dash for Your Calories

In chapter 5 you will learn how to calculate your calorie needs. The following table shows you how to find the DASH diet food plan that matches your personal calorie needs.

Unfortunately, many women, especially if they are short, need to be on a 1200 - 1600 calorie plan in order to lose weight. To give more flexibility for the lower calorie ranges, I have reduced the DASH portion sizes for fruits. This way you can include a more servings of fruit (just slightly smaller). Usually, a diet with more variety will make it easier to include the key DASH nutrients. And variety makes it easier to stay on a plan.

DASH Diet Calorie Adjustments				
	1200	1600	2000	2400

Fruits
  4 oz servings
  6 oz servings
	3 - 4	4 - 5	4 - 5	4 - 5

Vegetables	3 - 4	4 - 5	4 - 5	5 or more
Low fat and nonfat dairy	2 - 3	3	3	3 - 4
Beans and nuts	3 - 4 per week	3 - 4 per week	4 - 5 per week	5 per week
Lean meats, fish, poultry	5 oz	5 oz	7 oz	9 oz
Whole grains	3	3	3	3 - 5
Refined grains	0	3	5 - 6	6 - 8
Fats and sweets	2	3	4	5

Dash Tips for Intuitive Eaters

This section will give you quick tips to make specific changes in your diet to get all the benefits of the DASH diet, without having to think too much about the specifics. Want a complete menu plan? See chapter 3. Want to learn how to follow the DASH diet while you are eating in restaurants? See chapter 4.

1. **Double up.** The easiest way to be sure to get enough of the key DASH foods is to double up. (This is especially good if you tend to overeat, since it has you filling up on the best foods.) Instead of one 8-ounce glass of milk at breakfast, make it a 16-ounce glass, and you will have just had 2 servings of dairy. One cup of vegetables makes 2 servings. One cup of green beans, one small salad, and one cup of potatoes gives you 5 servings of vegetables at one meal.

2. **Don't double up.** (Sorry for the schizophrenic advice, there is something here for all sides of your personality.) Watch portions sizes where the calories may mount up quickly and where the foods aren't filling. Juices are one food item you don't want to double up. A large glass of juice has 240 Calories, little fiber, and won't keep you feeling full for very long. Limit juice to one serving per day. A DASH serving of juice is 6 ounces. Get the rest of your fruits and vegetables from whole foods, and you will stay full longer and find it easier to get to and maintain your healthy weight.

3. **Seek out DASH foods.** It's almost like a treasure hunt. Scan menus to find the DASH foods. When you go out to lunch or dinner, keep thinking, "How can I add extra fruits or vegetables." Add a serving of steamed vegetables to dinners and lunches. Choose to have your pasta sauce on vegetables rather than on pasta. Choose the diced fruit that is often offered as a french fry substitute. Add a salad if the restaurant is vegetable-challenged. At the very least you can add a glass of skim milk.

4. **Stockpile.** Keep your refrigerator and freezer stocked with DASH delights. Buy lots of bags of frozen foods at one time. Keep them fresh by using a clip-tight seal. Buy small portions of cut up fruit from the salad bar, if you buy what you will eat in 1 - 2 days, you won't have any waste.

5. **Can you find the hidden DASH foods?** Bring your sandwich to work, and top with grated carrots, shredded red cabbage, and sliced cucumber. Hide a glass of skim milk in your latte. Make your own pureed vegetable soup, take a thermos to work and drink your veggies.

6. **Buy convenience foods that just happen to be healthy foods.** We all know about bagged lettuce. But how about bagged carrot slices, broccoli or cauliflower tops, broccoli slaw (also known as confetti slaw), etc. Yogurt smoothies without the extra sugar. Milk chugs.

7. **Keep fresh foods fresh.** Use the new plastic bags that keep foods fresher longer. You are more

likely to buy fruits and vegetables if you don't
have to worry about them deteriorating before
you have a chance to use them. And you have
ready to eat fresh foods on a regular basis.

Keeping Track

Especially at the beginning, most of us need to
keep track of our servings, to see if we are really
meeting the DASH guidelines. On the following
page is an example of the DASH diet tracking form
which can help to keep you focused. Mark your goal
for the number of servings of each food group on the
bottom, and then check off each serving you
consume during the day. This will show your
progress in reaching your goals. You can find
downloadable larger sized versions of this form on
our web site at http://DASHdiet.org/forms.htm.

DASH Servings Check Off

	Monday	Tuesday	Wednesday	Thursday	Friday	Saturday	Sunday
Grains/starches: 1 slice bread; 1/2 cup cooked pasta, cereal, corn, potatoes; 1/3 c rice, 1 oz dry cereal; 1/4 bagel; 1/2 English muffin, bun; 2 cups popcorn, 2 small cookies	☐☐☐☐☐ ☐☐	☐☐☐☐☐ ☐☐	☐☐☐☐☐ ☐☐	☐☐☐☐☐ ☐☐	☐☐☐☐☐ ☐☐	☐☐☐☐☐ ☐☐	☐☐☐☐☐ ☐☐
Fruits: 4 oz juice, medium fruit, 1/4 cup dried fruit, 1/2 c canned fruit, 1 c large diced raw fruit	☐☐☐☐☐ ☐	☐☐☐☐☐ ☐	☐☐☐☐☐ ☐	☐☐☐☐☐ ☐	☐☐☐☐☐	☐☐☐☐☐ ☐	☐☐☐☐☐ ☐
Vegetables: 1/2 c cooked vegetables, 1 c leafy greens, 6 oz vegetable juice	☐☐☐☐☐ ☐	☐☐☐☐☐ ☐	☐☐☐☐☐ ☐	☐☐☐☐☐	☐☐☐☐☐	☐☐☐☐☐ ☐	☐☐☐☐☐ ☐
Low fat dairy: 8 oz skim or low fat milk, 8 oz low fat/fat-free yogurt, 1oz reduced fat cheese, 1/2 c fat free or low fat cottage cheese	☐☐☐☐☐	☐☐☐☐☐	☐☐☐☐☐	☐☐☐☐☐	☐☐☐☐☐	☐☐☐☐☐	☐☐☐☐☐
Beans, nuts, seeds: 1/4 c beans, nuts, seeds	☐☐☐☐☐	☐☐☐☐☐	☐☐☐☐☐	☐☐☐☐☐	☐☐☐☐☐	☐☐☐☐☐	☐☐☐☐☐
Lean meat, fish, poultry, eggs: Each ☐ = 1 oz. 1 egg = 1 oz, 2 egg whites = 1 oz	☐☐☐☐☐ ☐☐☐ ☐	☐☐☐☐☐ ☐☐☐ ☐	☐☐☐☐☐ ☐☐☐	☐☐☐☐☐ ☐☐☐	☐☐☐☐☐ ☐☐☐	☐☐☐☐☐ ☐☐☐ ☐	☐☐☐☐☐ ☐☐☐ ☐
Fats: 1 T salad dressing; 1 t butter, oil	☐☐☐☐☐	☐☐☐☐☐	☐☐☐☐☐	☐☐☐☐☐	☐☐☐☐☐	☐☐☐☐☐	☐☐☐☐☐
Water, liquids: 8 ounces	☐☐☐☐☐ ☐☐☐	☐☐☐☐☐ ☐☐☐	☐☐☐☐☐ ☐☐☐	☐☐☐☐☐ ☐☐☐	☐☐☐☐☐ ☐☐☐	☐☐☐☐☐ ☐☐☐	☐☐☐☐☐ ☐☐☐

Grains/starches _____
Fruits _____
Vegetables _____

Dairy _____
Beans/nuts _____
Meats, fish, poultry _____

Fats _____
Fluid _____

© 2004, Marla Heller, MS, RD

Chapter 2 DASHboard

1. Double up on low cal DASH when you have the chance, especially non-starchy vegetables and low fat or nonfat dairy.
2. Limit portion sizes on higher calorie foods.
3. Stock your cupboards and fridge with the key DASH diet foods.
4. Sneak in extra DASH foods. Toss extra raw veggies in your sandwich or have a latte with 8 oz skim milk.
5. Buy DASH convenience foods, such as bagged pre-cut veggies, yogurt smoothies, and single-serve bottles of milk.

Tracking my Personal DASH Diet Action Plan:
Specific changes I will make in my diet include:

_____

_____

_____

_____

I will track my intake by using:

_____, _____ days per week.

Chapter 3 2000 Calorie DASH Menus for 28 Days

This chapter provides you with 28 days of menus for a 2000 calorie diet, with adjustments for 1200 and 1600 calories. If your calorie needs are different, you can use the guidelines in chapter 2 to find out how to reduce (or increase) the calories as needed. Chapter 5 provides information on how to calculate your calorie needs, which is especially important if you are trying to lose weight.

Where appropriate, serving sizes refer to cooked portions, all weight measures are noted as oz (ounces), and liquid measures are noted as fl oz (fluid ounces), t (teaspoon), T (tablespoon) and c (cup). For example 6 ounces of strawberries will be more than a cup (depending on the size and if they are sliced), while 6 fluid ounces of orange juice is the volume you would get from a measuring cup. I recommend using a digital kitchen scale to help you get the idea of serving sizes for the DASH diet (and to help with managing your weight).

Many of the menus include recipes that are located in chapter 14. These recipes are indicated by being written in italics, followed by an asterisk, as in *chicken cacciatore**.

These menus meet or exceed the DASH guidelines. The menus were designed to provide 2000 calories, have less than 30% fat, less than 7% saturated fat, less than 200 mg cholesterol, at least 25 grams of fiber, less than 1750 mg sodium, greater than 4000 mg potassium, greater than 1200 mg calcium, and greater than 400 mg magnesium. The diet plan meets or exceeds all other RDA values for vitamins and minerals for people over the age of 50.

The following menus have adjustments for 1200 and 1600 calorie diets. Any needed adjustments for 1200 calories are in parentheses, and any 1600 calorie modifications are in brackets. For example, on the next page, someone following a 1200 calorie plan would have 1 oz Wheaties with 4 oz strawberries, 4 oz juice, and 8 oz skim milk. The 1600 calorie plan would include all of the above and the toast and jam. In general, the lower calorie plans have 4 oz serving sizes of fruits (small versus medium), 1 T of regular salad dressings, 1 T of nuts, 0.6 oz cheeses, and 2 oz meat, fish, or poultry at lunch and 3 oz at dinner. Usually the 1200 calorie plan is limited in desserts (sigh . . .).

Week 1

Monday 2000 [1600] (1200) Calories
Breakfast
Cereal, Strawberries, OJ, Toast, and Milk
1 oz Wheaties, topped with 6 oz strawberries [(4 oz)]
6 fl oz orange juice [(4 fl oz)]
1 slice whole wheat toast (0) , with 2 t strawberry jam (0)
8 fl oz nonfat milk

Lunch
Half Tuna Sandwich, Side Salad, Nectarine, Milk
half tuna sandwich: 1 slice wheat berry bread (0) , with 1/2 c
    low sodium, light tuna salad* [(1/3 c)], topped with 1/4 c
    cucumber slices
side salad: 1 c romaine lettuce, with 8 grape tomatoes, and 2 T
    nonfat Italian dressing, with no added salt
8 fl oz nonfat milk
1 medium nectarine [(small)]

Snack
Almonds and Yogurt
1/4 c almonds [(1 T)]
6 oz nonfat, artificially sweetened peach yogurt

Dinner
Chicken Piccata, Potatoes, Haricots Verts, Green Salad,
    Chocolate Chip Cookies, Grapes
3 oz *chicken piccata**
1 serving *Parmesan potatoes** (0)
1/2 c haricots verts (skinny french green beans)
green salad: 1 1/2 c mixed greens, topped with 2 T oil and
    vinegar dressing [(1 T)]
2 chocolate chip cookies [(0)]
1 c grapes (0)

DASH servings: 5 vegetables, 3 fruit, 3 dairy, 1 nuts, 3 whole
grains, 1 refined grain, 6 oz meats

Week 1 Tuesday 2000 [1600] (1200) Calories

Breakfast
Omelette, Toast, Mixed Berries, Peach Nectar, and Latte
1 *Southwestern egg white omelette** [(1/2)]
2 slices whole wheat toast (0) [1] , topped with 4 t raspberry
    jam (0) [2 t]
1 c mixed blueberries, strawberries, and raspberries
6 fl oz peach nectar [(4 fl oz)]
coffee latte: 8 fl oz nonfat milk and 2 fl oz espresso

Lunch
Ham and Swiss Sandwich, Raw Veggies, Apple
ham and Swiss sandwich: 2 slices whole grain bread [(1)] , 2 oz
    ham, and 1 oz low sodium, low fat Swiss cheese [(0.6)],
    topped with 1/4 c shredded cabbage, 2 slices tomato, and
    mustard
1/2 c carrots "chips" (crinkle-cut raw carrot chips)
8 grape tomatoes
1 medium Granny Smith apple [(small)]

Snack
Hazelnuts, Cantaloupe, Yogurt
1/4 c hazelnuts [(1 T)]
4 oz cantaloupe
6 oz nonfat, artificially sweetened strawberry-kiwi yogurt

Dinner
Salmon on a Bed of Mashed Sweet Potato with Broccoli,
    Mesclun Salad, Bread, Frozen Yogurt
4 oz grilled salmon [(3 oz)]
1/2 c mashed sweet potato
1 c steamed broccoli
mesclun salad: 11/2 c mixed baby greens, topped with 2 T
    champaign vinaigrette dressing [(1 T)]
1 slice Italian bread (0)
1/2 c nonfat, artificially sweetened frozen yogurt

DASH servings: 4 whole grain, 1 refined grain, 3 dairy, 4 fruit,
5+ vegetables, 1 nuts, 8 oz meats

24

Week 1 Wednesday 2000 [1600] (1200) Calories

Breakfast
French Toast Topped with Sliced Canned Peaches, Strawberry-
Banana Smoothie
2 slices whole wheat French toast [(1)], topped with 1/2 c sliced
peaches [(1/4 c)]
smoothie: 4 oz strawberries, 1/2 banana, and 8 fl oz nonfat
milk

Lunch
· Open Face Tuna Melt, Oven Fries, Coleslaw, Peas and Carrots,
Milk, Apple
open face tuna melt: 1/2 c *low sodium tuna salad** [(1/3 c)], with
1 oz low sodium, low fat cheddar cheese [(0.6 oz)], on 1 slice
whole wheat bread
1 serving *oven potato fries** (1/2 serving)
1 c coleslaw [(1/2 c)]
1/2 c peas and carrots
8 fl oz nonfat milk
1 medium Fuji apple [(small)]

Snack
Baby Carrots Dipped in Spreadable Cheese, Almonds
8 baby carrots dipped in 1 Light Laughing Cow™ Spreadable
Cheese
1/4 c almonds [(1 T)]

Dinner
Pollo Alla Grilglia on a Bed of Mixed Baby Greens, Grape
Tomatoes, and Roasted Potatoes, with Steamed Spinach,
and Mixed Berries and Plums
*Pollo alla griglia** on a bed of 1 1/2 c mixed baby greens, 8 grape
tomatoes, 1/2 c roasted potatoes, and 2 T oil and vinegar
dressing [(1 T)]
1/2 c steamed spinach
1 c mixed raspberries, sliced plums, and blueberries [(1/2 c)]

DASH servings: 3 whole grain, 4 fruits, 6 vegetables, 3 dairy, 1
nuts, 6 ounces meats

Week 1 Thursday 2000 [1600] (1200) Calories

Breakfast
Quick Scramblers, Sliced Strawberries, Toast, OJ, and Milk
Quick Scramblers: In microwave-safe dish, sprayed with
    nonstick cooking spray, microwave 1/2 c Egg Beaters™
    Southwestern Style [(1/4 c)], 2 minutes on high.
6 oz sliced strawberries [(4 oz)]
1 slice whole wheat toast (0), topped with 2 t strawberry
    preserves (0)
6 fl oz orange juice [(4 fl oz)]
8 fl oz nonfat milk

Lunch
Beef and Swiss Sandwich, Potato Chips, Grape Tomatoes, Milk,
Pluot
lean beef and Swiss sandwich: 2 slices whole wheat bread [(1)],
    2 oz lean beef , 1 oz low sodium, low fat Swiss cheese [(0.6)],
    topped with 1/4 c shredded romaine lettuce, 2 slices of
    tomato, and mustard
1 oz lightly salted baked potato chips [(0)]
8 grape tomatoes
8 fl oz nonfat milk
1 pluot (a delicious cross between a plum and an apricot)

Snack
Apple Slices Dipped in Peanut Butter
apple slices from 1 medium apple [(small)], dipped in 2 T
    natural peanut butter [(1 T)]

Dinner
Lean, Meaty Spaghetti, Green Beans, Dinner Salad, and Frozen
    Yogurt
spaghetti with extra lean meat sauce: 1 c *Lean, Meaty spaghetti
    sauce** on 1 c spaghetti (½ c)
1/2 c green beans
dinner salad: 1 1/2 c green salad, topped with 2 T nonfat
    Italian dressing, with no added salt
1/2 c nonfat, artificially sweetened frozen yogurt (0)

Dash servings: 3 whole grains, 4 fruits, 5 vegetables, 3+ dairy, 1
nuts, 7 oz meats

Week 1 Friday 2000 [1600] (1200) Calories

Breakfast
Mini Muffins, Yogurt, OJ, and Milk
2 orange-cranberry mini muffins [(1)]
6 oz nonfat, artificially sweetened strawberry yogurt (0)
6 fl oz orange juice [(4 fl oz)]
8 fl oz nonfat milk

Lunch
Turkey, Swiss Rollup, Side Salad, and Peach
turkey, Swiss, cranberry rollup: 1 whole wheat flour tortilla
    [(1/2)], spread with 1/4 c cranberry sauce (1 T), layered
    with 3 oz turkey breast [(2 oz)] and 1 oz low fat Colby-jack
    cheese [(0.6 oz)]
side salad: 1 c greens and mixed vegetables topped with 1 T oil
    and vinegar dressing
1 medium peach [(small)]

Snack
Cottage Cheese, Walnuts, and Plum
4 oz cottage cheese, 1% fat, no salt added
1 medium plum [(small)]
1/4 c walnuts [(1 T)]

Dinner
Pork Chop with Baked Sweet Potato, Applesauce, Asparagus,
    and Dinner Salad
5 oz pork loin chop [(3 oz)]
1 c baked sweet potato (1/2)
1/2 c applesauce, unsweetened
1 c asparagus
dinner salad: 1 1/2 c lettuce and mixed vegetables, topped with
    2 T French dressing [(1 t)]

DASH servings: 1 whole grains, 4 fruits, 6+ vegetables, 3+
dairy, 1 nuts, 8 oz meats

Week 1 Saturday 2000 [1600] (1200) Calories

Breakfast
English Muffin with Cheese, Melon, Orange-tangerine Juice,
    and Milk
1 cinnamon- raisin English muffin (1/2), topped with
    1 Light Laughing Cow Creamy Spreadable Cheese
6 oz honeydew melon [(4 oz)]
6 fl oz orange tangerine juice [(4 fl oz)]
8 fl oz nonfat milk

Lunch
Colorful Beef Tacos and Peach
3 taco shells[(2)], filled with 3 oz *extra lean taco filling** [(2 oz)]
    and topped with 1 oz low sodium, low fat cheddar cheese
    [(0.6 oz)], diced red tomatoes, shredded romaine lettuce,
    shredded carrots, and shredded red cabbage
1 medium peach [(small)]

Snack
Apple, Popcorn, and Cheese
1 medium apple [(small)]
2 c popcorn (0)
1 light string cheese

Dinner
Steak, Baked Potato, Broccoli, Salad
4 oz broiled T-bone steak [(3 oz)]
baked potato (0)
1/2 c broccoli
dinner salad: 1 1/2 c greens and mixed vegetables, topped with
    2 T Thousand Island dressing [(1 T)]
1 slice whole wheat bread [(0)], topped with 1 t soft, unsalted
margarine [(0)]
6 oz nonfat, artificially sweetened peach yogurt

DASH servings: 5 whole grains, 4 fruits, 5 vegetables, 3+ dairy,
1 nuts, 7 oz meats

Week 1 Sunday 2000 [1600] (1200) Calories

Breakfast
Egg white omelette, with Bagel, Cheese, OJ, and Milk
egg white omelette
1/2 poppy seed bagel, topped with Laughing Cow™ Light
    Creamy French Onion Spreadable Cheese
6 fl oz fresh squeezed orange juice [(4 fl oz)]
8 fl oz nonfat milk

Lunch
Grilled Cheese with Tomato, Cucumber Salad, Peaches
grilled cheese: 2 slices whole grain bread (1), 1 oz low sodium,
    low fat Swiss cheese (0.6 oz) , 2 slices tomato (1)
3/4 c sliced cucumber topped with 1 T nonfat, no added salt,
    Italian dressing
1 cup sliced peaches, canned in juice [(1/2 c)]

Snack
Yogurt, Peanuts, and Cantaloupe
6 oz nonfat, artificially sweetened vanilla yogurt
1/4 c peanuts, dry roasted, unsalted [(1 T)]
6 oz cantaloupe [4 oz] (0)

Dinner
Roasted Chicken with Potatoes, Carrots, and Brussels Sprouts,
    Pudding and Pear
1 serving *roasted chicken with potatoes, carrots and Brussels
    sprouts**
1/2 c chocolate pudding (0)
1 medium pear [(small)]

DASH servings: 2 whole grains, 5 fruits, 5+ vegetables, 3+
dairy, 1 nuts, 8 oz meats

Week 2

Week 2 Monday 2000 [1600] (1200) Calories

Breakfast
Scrambled Eggs, Toast, Pineapple, OJ, and Milk
quick scramblers: in microwave-safe dish, sprayed with
    nonstick cooking spray, cook 1/2 c egg substitutes [(1/4 c)],
    approximately 3 [(2)] minutes on high.
2 slices whole wheat toast [(1)], topped with 4 t orange
marmalade [(2 t)]
6 oz pineapple [(4 oz)]
6 fl oz orange juice [(4 fl oz)]
8 fl oz nonfat milk

Lunch
Chicken Waldorf salad, with Roll, Italian Cole Slaw, Milk, and
Strawberry Gelatin
1/2 c *chicken Waldorf salad** (1/3 c)
1 whole wheat dinner roll
1 c *Italian cole slaw** [(1/4 c)]
8 fl oz nonfat milk
1/2 c artificially sweetened strawberry gelatin
1 medium plum [(small)]

Snack
Banana and Yogurt
1 medium banana [(small)]
6 oz nonfat, artificially sweetened strawberry-banana yogurt

Dinner
Grilled Tilapia with Potatoes, Asparagus, Salad, and Frozen
    Yogurt
3 oz grilled tilapia
1 c potatoes (1/2 c)
1 c asparagus
dinner salad: 1 1/2 c greens and mixed vegetables, topped with
    2 T oil and vinegar dressing [(1 T)]
1 c artificially sweetened, nonfat strawberry frozen yogurt (1/2 c)

DASH servings: 3 whole grains, 4+ fruits, 6 vegetables, 4 dairy,
8 oz meats

Week 2 Tuesday 2000 [1600] (1200) Calories

Breakfast
English Muffin, PB, Yogurt, Orange, and Milk
1 mixed grain English muffin [(1/2)], topped with
    1 T natural peanut butter, no salt added [(2 t)]
6 oz nonfat, artificially sweetened strawberry banana yogurt
1 medium orange [(small)]
8 fl oz nonfat milk

Lunch
Veggie Burger, with Fries, Coleslaw, and Banana
veggie burger: whole wheat hamburger bun (0) with grilled
    vegetable burger patty, soy based, topped with 1 oz low
    sodium, low fat Swiss cheese [(0.6)], 2 slices red tomato, 1/4
    c shredded romaine lettuce
1 serving oven potato fries* (1/2)
1/2 c coleslaw (1/4)
1 medium banana [(small)]

Snack
Cottage Cheese, Pear, and Walnuts
4 oz cottage cheese, no salt added, 1% fat
1 medium pear [(small)]
1/4 c walnuts [(1 T)]

Dinner
Roast Chicken Breast, Baked Potato, Honey Glazed Carrots,
    Salad, and Frozen Yogurt
4 oz roasted chicken breast [(3 oz)]
baked potato (1/2)
1 c honey-glazed carrots
dinner salad: 1 1/2 c greens and mixed vegetables, topped with
    2 T Italian dressing [(1 T)]
1/2 c artificially sweetened, nonfat chocolate frozen yogurt (0)

DASH servings: 4 whole grains, 3 fruits, 6+ vegetables, 4 dairy,
1 beans, 1 nuts, 4 oz meats

Week 2 Wednesday 2000 [1600] (1200) Calories

Breakfast
Oatmeal and Sliced Banana, Whole Wheat Toast, Red
Grapefruit, and Milk
1/2 c instant oatmeal, unsweetened, topped with 1
    sliced banana [(1/2)]
1 slice whole wheat toast (0), topped with
    2 t strawberry preserves (0)
6 oz red grapefruit [(4 oz)]
8 fl oz nonfat milk

Lunch
Soup, Cheese & Crackers, Side Salad, Yogurt, and Apple
1 c low sodium vegetable beef soup (3/4 c)
1 oz low sodium, low fat Swiss cheese [(0.6 oz)], with
    6 low salt whole wheat crackers (4)
side salad: 1 c greens and mixed vegetables, topped with
    2 T buttermilk ranch dressing [(1 T)]
6 oz nonfat, artificially sweetened peach yogurt
1 medium apple [(small)]

Snack
Cheese and a Peach
1 piece light string cheese
1 medium peach [(small)]

Dinner
Pork Chop, Scalloped Potatoes, Green Beans, Carrot- Raisin
    Salad, Walnuts, and Milk
4 oz broiled pork loin chop [(3 oz)]
1/2 c scalloped potatoes
1 c green beans
1/2 c carrot raisin salad (1/4 c), mixed with 1/4 c walnuts [(1
T)]
8 fl oz nonfat milk

DASH servings: 3 whole grains, 4 fruits, 7 vegetables, 4+ dairy,
1 nuts, 4 oz meats

Week 2 Thursday 2000 [1600] (1200) Calories

Breakfast
Cereal, Cantaloupe, Orange Juice, and Milk
1 1/2 oz raisin bran cereal
6 oz cantaloupe [(4 oz)]
6 fl oz orange juice [(4 fl oz)]
8 fl oz nonfat milk

Lunch
Grilled Cheese, Side Salad, Raw Veggies, and Pear
grilled cheese with tomato, made with 2 slice(s) whole grain
    bread, 1 oz low sodium, low fat cheddar cheese, and 2 slices
    tomato
side salad: 1 c greens and mixed vegetables, topped with 2 T
    french dressing [1 T] (2 T fat free dressing)
8 baby carrots
2 celery stalks
1 medium pear [(small)]

Snack
Strawberry Smoothie and Almonds
smoothie: 8 fl oz nonfat milk and 6 oz strawberries [(4 oz)]
1/4 c almonds [(1 T)]

Dinner
Carribean Chicken, Rice, Cheesy Broccoli, and Salad
1 serving *Carribean chicken**
1 c long grain white rice (0)
Cheesy broccoli: 1/2 c broccoli, topped with melted 1 oz low
    sodium, low fat cheddar cheese [(0.6)]
dinner salad: 1 1/2 c greens and mixed vegetables, topped with
    2 T honey mustard dressing [(1 T)]

DASH servings: 3 whole grains, 5 fruits, 5 vegetables, 3 dairy, 1
nuts, 7 oz meats

Week 2 Friday 2000 [1600] (1200) Calories

Breakfast
Cereal, Banana, Milk, Juice
1 oz Cheerios™ topped with sliced banana [(1/2)]
6 fl oz orange strawberry banana juice [(4 fl oz)]
8 fl oz nonfat milk

Lunch
Tuna in a Pita, Side Salad, Grapes
tuna pita: 1/2 whole wheat pita bread (0), 1/2 c *low sodium tuna salad** (1/3 c), 2 slices red tomato, handful of radish sprouts
side salad: 1 c greens and mixed vegetables, topped with 2 T blue cheese dressing with Roquefort cheese [(1 T)]
6 oz grapes [(4 oz)]

Snack
Peanuts and Plum
1/4 c peanuts, dry roasted, unsalted [(1 T)]
1 medium plum [(small)]

Dinner
Cheeseburger, Coleslaw, Veggies, Sundae
extra lean cheeseburger: 4 oz 95% lean ground beef [(3 oz)], topped with 1 oz low sodium, low fat Swiss cheese [(0.6 oz)], 2 slices tomato, and lettuce on a hamburger bun
1/2 c coleslaw (1/4 c)
1 c broccoli, carrots, and cauliflower
sundae: 1 c raspberries [3/4 c] (½ c) on 6 oz nonfat, artificially sweetened vanilla yogurt

DASH servings: 2 whole grains, 4 fruits, 4+ vegetables, 3 dairy, 1 nuts, 7 oz meats

Week 2 Saturday 2000 [1600] (1200) Calories

Breakfast
Bagel with Cheese, Strawberries, Hot Chocolate, and OJ
1/2 whole grain bagel spread with 1 Light Laughing Cow
    Creamy Spreadable Cheese™
6 oz strawberries [(4 oz)]
hot chocolate: 8 fl oz nonfat milk, 1 heaping teaspoon dry
    cocoa, and 2 packages of Splenda™
6 fl oz orange juice [(4 fl oz)]

Lunch
Bean and Cheese Burrito, Side Salad, and Pear
1 bean and cheese burrito (1/2), topped with 1/4 oz shredded
    low sodium Colby cheese, topped with 4 oz mango salsa
1/2 cup Mexicali corn
side salad: 1 c lettuce salad with tomatoes and carrots, topped
    with 1 T pine nuts, and 1 T oil and vinegar dressing
1 medium pear [(small)]

Snack
Latte, Cookies, and Fruit Salad
coffee latte, made with 8 fl oz nonfat milk and 2 fl oz espresso
2 sugar cookies
1/2 c fruit salad [(0)]

Dinner
New York Strip Steak, Asparagus, Dinner Salad, Peach-Apple
    Crisp
4 oz New York strip steak [(3 oz)]
1 c asparagus
dinner salad: 1 1/2 c greens and mixed vegetables, topped with
    2 T oil and vinegar dressing [(1 T)]
1/2 c peach apple crisp, topped with 1/2 c nonfat, artificially
    sweetened vanilla frozen yogurt [1/4 c] (0)

DASH servings: 3 whole grains, 5 fruits, 5 vegetables, 5 dairy, 1
beans, 1 nuts, 4 oz meats

Week 2 Sunday 2000 [1600] (1200) Calories

Breakfast
California Scramble, Pineapple, Latte, and OJ
California scramble: 1 whole wheat flour tortilla (1/2)], filled
    with 1/2 c scrambled egg substitutes (1/4 c), topped with 3
    avocado slices (2), and 2 oz salsa
6 oz pineapple [(4 oz)]
coffee latte: 2 fl oz espresso, and 8 fl oz nonfat milk
6 fl oz orange juice [(4 fl oz)]

Lunch
Roast Beef and Swiss on Rye
roast beef and Swiss on rye: 3 oz lean roast beef [(2 oz)], 1 oz
    low sodium, low fat Swiss cheese [(0.6)], on 2 slices rye
    bread (1) with mustard
8 baby carrots
6 radishes
side salad: 1 c greens and mixed vegetables, topped with 2 T oil
    and vinegar dressing [(1 T)]
8 fl oz nonfat milk
1 medium peach [(small)]

Snack
Tomato Bisque with Crackers and Tangerine
3/4 c low sodium tomato bisque soup (1/2 c) with 6 low salt
    whole wheat crackers (2)
1 medium tangerine [(small)]

Dinner
Pile It On! Chili and Sundae
1 c *Pile It On! chili** (3/4 c), topped with 1 oz low sodium, low
    fat cheddar cheese [(0.6)], 2 T fat free sour cream, and *baked
    corn tortilla strips**
sundae: 1/2 c nonfat, artificially sweetened frozen yogurt,
    topped with 6 oz raspberries [(4 oz)]

DASH servings: 3 whole grains, 6 fruits, 4 vegetables, 3+ dairy,
1 nuts, 7 oz meats

Week 3

Week 3 Monday 2000 [1600] (1200) Calories

Breakfast
1 oz Special K, topped with 6 oz strawberries [(4 oz)]
1 slice whole wheat toast, topped with 2 t strawberry jam
6 fl oz freshly squeezed orange juice [(4 fl oz)]
8 fl oz nonfat milk

Lunch
Turkey and Swiss on Rye, Carrots, Coleslaw, and Orange
turkey and Swiss on rye: 3 oz roasted turkey breast [(2 oz)], 1
    oz low sodium, low fat Swiss cheese [(0.6)] on 2 slices rye
    bread [(1)]
1 c sliced carrots
1 c coleslaw [1/2 c] (1/4 c)
1 medium navel orange [(small)]

Snack
Gelatin, Cottage Cheese, and Nectarine
1/2 c artificially sweetened strawberry gelatin
4 oz cottage cheese, no salt added, 1% fat
1 medium nectarine [(small)

Dinner
Lean, Meaty Spaghetti, Asparagus, Salad, Wine, and Frozen
Yogurt
1 c *lean, meaty spaghetti sauce* [(3/4 c)]* on 1 1/2 c spaghetti [(1 c)]
1 c asparagus
dinner salad: 1 1/2 c greens and mixed vegetables, topped with
    2 T oil and vinegar dressing [(1 T)]
4 fl oz red wine [(0)]
1/2 c nonfat, artificially sweetened frozen yogurt (0)

DASH servings: 4 whole grains, 4 fruits, 6+ vegetables, 3 dairy,
6 oz meats

Week 3 Tuesday 2000 [1600] (1200) Calories

Breakfast
Cereal, English Muffin, Honeydew, OJ, and Milk
1 oz Honey Nut Cheerios™
1/2 raisin and cinnamon English muffin (0), topped with 1 t
    soft margarine, unsalted (0)
6 oz honeydew [(4 oz)]
6 oz orange juice [(4 fl oz)]
8 fl oz nonfat milk

Lunch
Tuna and Swiss Sandwich, Salad, and Peach
tuna salad & Swiss Sandwich: 1/2 c *low sodium tuna salad** [(1/3
    c)], 1 oz low sodium, low fat Swiss cheese [(0.6 oz)], on 2
    slices whole wheat bread [(1)]
side Salad: 1 c greens and mixed vegetables, topped with 2 T
    Thousand Island dressing [(1 T)]
1 medium peach [(small)]

Snack
Yogurt, Pecans, and Strawberries
6 oz nonfat, artificially sweetened strawberry kiwi yogurt
1/4 c pecans, unsalted [(1 T)]
6 oz strawberries [(4 oz)]

Dinner
Pasta e Fagioli alla Venezia, Caprese Salad, and Pears
Pasta e Fagioli alla Venezia* (1/2 serving)
Caprese salad: 1 oz sliced fresh mozzarella [(0.6 oz)] alternated
    with the slices of 1 tomato, dressed with 1 T extra virgin
    olive oil and 1 T balsamic vinegar, dusted with, 1 leaf fresh
    basil, cut into thin strips
1/2 c sliced Bartlett pears

DASH servings: 3 whole grains, 5 fruits, 3 vegetables, 4 dairy, 1
nuts, 1 beans, 3 oz meats

Week 3 Wednesday 2000 [1600] (1200) Calories

. *Breakfast*
Blueberry Muffin, Cheese, Cantaloupe, Juice, and Milk
1 small blueberry muffin
1 piece light string cheese
6 oz cantaloupe [(4 oz)]
6 fl oz orange tangerine juice [(4 fl oz)]
8 fl oz nonfat milk

Lunch
Lean Cheeseburger, Coleslaw, Veggies, and Apple
cheeseburger: 3 oz extra lean ground sirloin [(2 oz)], broiled,
    topped with 1 oz reduced fat, reduced sodium Swiss cheese
    [(0.6 oz)], on a whole wheat hamburger bun, with 1 t yellow
    mustard, 1 t catsup or ketchup
1/2 c coleslaw (1/4 c)
1/2 c broccoli and carrots
1 medium Golden Delicious apple [(small)]

Snack
Raw Pepper Strips Dipped in Guacamole
1 c sliced bell pepper strips, dipped in
    4 T guacamole (2 T)

Dinner
Peach-Mustard Glazed Pork Chop, Sweet Potato, Peas, Salad,
and Yogurt Topped with Mixed Berries
peach-mustard glazed pork chop* [(3 oz)]
1 c baked sweet potato (1/2 c)
1 c green peas (1/2 c)
dinner salad: 1 1/2 c greens and mixed vegetables, topped with
    2 T oil and vinegar dressing [(1 T)]
1 c nonfat, artificially sweetened frozen vanilla yogurt [(1/2 c)],
    topped with 1 c mixed raspberries and blackberries [(1/2 c)]

DASH servings: 2 whole grains, 4 fruits, 7 vegetables, 4 dairy, 6
oz meats

Week 3 Thursday 2000 [1600] (1200) Calories

Breakfast
Oatmeal with Applesauce, Yogurt, Juice, and English Muffin
1/2 c oatmeal, mixed with 1/2 c applesauce [(1/4 c)],
    unsweetened, and sprinkled with cinnamon
1/2 whole wheat English muffin (0), topped with 1 t raspberry jam (0)
6 oz nonfat, artificially sweetened vanilla yogurt
6 fl oz pineapple juice [(4 fl oz)]

Lunch
Chicken Waldorf Salad Topped with Walnuts, Roll, Carrots,
    Milk, and Cantaloupe
1/2 c chicken Waldorf salad [(1/3 c)], topped with 1 T chopped
    walnuts
1 small whole wheat dinner roll (0)
8 baby carrots
1 c Italian cole slaw [1/2 c] (1/4 c)
8 fl oz nonfat milk
6 oz cantaloupe [(4 oz)]

Snack
Cheese and Kiwi
1 piece light string cheese
2 kiwifruit (1)

Dinner
Roasted Chicken Breast, Baked Potato, Asparagus, Tomato
    Spinach Salad, and Apple Crisp
4 oz roasted chicken breast [(3 oz)]
1/2 medium baked sweet potato
1 c asparagus
tomato spinach salad: 1 c baby spinach, 1 tomato, wedged,
    drizzled with 1 T olive oil and balsamic vinegar
apple crisp [(0)], topped with 1/2 c nonfat, artificially
    sweetened vanilla frozen yogurt (0)

DASH servings: 3 whole grains, 5 fruits, 6 vegetables, 3 dairy,
1/2 nuts, 7 oz meats

40

Week 3 Friday 2000 [1600] (1200) Calories

Breakfast
Chocolate Glazed Doughnut, Banana, OJ, and Latte
chocolate glazed cake doughnut
banana (1/2)
6 fl oz orange juice [(4 fl oz)]
Coffee latte: 2 fl oz espresso and 8 fl oz nonfat milk

Lunch
Veggie Dog, Chips, Cucumber Salad, Veggies, Milk, and
. Watermelon
veggie dog: whole wheat hot dog bun, soy based veggie hot
    dog, topped with yellow mustard
1 oz no salt potato chips [(0)]
1/2 c cucumber slices, dipped in 2 T ranch dressing [(1 T)]
8 baby carrots
8 grape tomatoes
8 fl oz nonfat milk
6 oz watermelon [(4 oz)]

Snack
Apple Dipped in PB
1 medium apple [(small)], slices dipped in 2 T natural peanut
    butter [(1 T)]

Dinner
Veggie-Cheese Pizza, Salad, and Trifle
2 slices cheese pizza (1), topped with green peppers, tomato,
    and mushrooms
dinner salad: 1 1/2 c greens and mixed vegetables, topped with
    2 T nonfat Italian dressing, no salt added
trifle: 1/2 c custard, topped with 1/4 c sliced strawberries and
    1/2 sliced banana (1/4), and 2 T whipped cream [(0)]

DASH servings: 2 whole grains, 5 fruits, 6 vegetables, 4 dairy, 1
nuts, 1 beans

Week 3 Saturday 2000 [1600] (1200) Calories

Breakfast
Waffles, Maple Syrup, Breakfast Patty, Banana, OJ, and Milk
2 low fat whole wheat waffles [(1)], topped with 1/4 c reduced
    calorie maple syrup [(2 T)]
1 veggie (soy-based) breakfast patty (0)
banana (1/2)
6 fl oz orange juice [(4 fl oz)]
8 fl oz nonfat milk

Lunch
Oriental Chicken Salad on Snow Pea Pods, Milk, and Plum
3/4 c oriental chicken salad [(1/2 c)] on a bed of 1 c snow pea
    pods
8 fl oz nonfat milk
1 medium plum [(small)]

Snack
Yogurt and Cashews
6 oz nonfat, artificially sweetened blueberry yogurt
1/4 c cashews, unsalted [(1 T)]

Dinner
Halibut in Balsamic Reduction, on a Bed of Smashed Red
    Potatoes, Brussels Sprouts, Salad, and Brownie
3 oz *halibut in balsamic reduction** on a bed of 1/2 c *smashed red
    potatoes** (0)
1 c Brussels sprouts
dinner salad: 1 1/2 c greens and mixed vegetables, topped with
    2 T oil and vinegar dressing [(1 T)]
brownie (0)

DASH servings: 2 whole grains, 3 fruits, 5 vegetables, 3 dairy, 1
nuts, 6 oz meats

Week 3 Sunday 2000 [1600] (1200) Calories

Breakfast
Bagel and cheese, Cereal, Blueberries, OJ, and Milk
1/2 sesame seed bagel (0), topped with 1 Light Laughing Cow
    Creamy Spreadable Cheese™ (0)
1 c Wheaties™
4 oz blueberries
6 fl oz orange juice [(4 fl oz)]
8 fl oz nonfat milk

Lunch
PB & J on Wheat, Chicken Noodle Soup, Milk, and Pineapple
PB & J: 2 slices whole wheat bread (1), 1 T natural peanut
    butter (2 t), 1 T grape jelly (2 t)
1 c low fat chicken noodle soup, no salt added [(3/4 c)]
8 fl oz nonfat milk
6 oz pineapple [(4 oz)]

Snack
Hot Chocolate and Strawberries
hot chocolate: 8 fl oz nonfat milk, 1 t unsweetened cocoa
    powder, and 2 packages of Splenda™
6 oz strawberries [(4 oz)]

Dinner
BBQ Beef Sandwich, Oven Fries, Sweet Corn, Italian Cole Slaw,
    and Chocolate Frozen Yogurt
BBQ sandwich: 1/2 c beef with barbecue sauce on a whole
    wheat hamburger bun [(0)]
1 serving *oven potato fries** [(1/2)]
1/2 c sweet corn
1 c Italian cole slaw [(1/2 c)]
1/2 c unsweetened applesauce
1/2 c nonfat, artificially sweetened frozen chocolate yogurt (0)

DASH servings: 5 whole grains, 6 fruits, 3+ vegetables, 3+
dairy, 1 nuts, 3 oz meats

Week 4

Week 4 Monday 2000 [1600] (1200) Calories

Breakfast
Cereal and Berries, Milk, OJ, and Toast
1 oz bran flakes, topped with 3 oz blackberries [(2 oz)] and 3 oz
    raspberries [(2 oz)]
8 fl oz nonfat milk
6 fl oz orange juice [(4 fl oz)]
1 slice whole wheat toast, topped with 2 t raspberry preserves

Lunch
Lean Roast Beef and Swiss on Rye, Cole Slaw, Milk, and
Cantaloupe
lean roast beef and Swiss: 3 oz lean roast beef [(2 oz)], 1 oz low
    sodium, low fat Swiss cheese [(0.6 oz)] on 2 slices rye bread [(1)]
1/2 c *Italian cole slaw** [1/2 c] (1/4 c)
8 fl oz nonfat milk
6 oz cantaloupe [(4 oz)]

Snack
Orange and Cashews
California navel orange
1/4 c cashews [(1 T)]

Dinner
Chicken Cacciatore, Potato Wedges, Peas, Salad, and Italian
    Bread
*chicken cacciatore**
4 oz potato wedges
1/2 c baby sweet peas.
dinner salad: 1 1/2 c greens and mixed vegetables, topped with
    2 T Italian dressing [(1 T)]
1 slice Italian bread (0), topped with 1 t soft, unsalted
    margarine (0)

DASH servings: 4 whole grains, 4 fruit, 4 vegetables, 4 dairy, 1
nuts, 6 oz meats

Week 4 Tuesday 2000 [1600] (1200) Calories

Breakfast
Blueberry Waffles, Honeydew, Juice, and Latte
2 blueberry waffles (1), topped with 2 T light maple syrup (1T)
6 oz honeydew [(4)]
6 fl oz grapefruit juice [(4 fl oz)]
latte: 8 fl oz nonfat milk and 2 fl oz espresso

Lunch
Cobb Salad, Roll, Milk, and Strawberries
1 1/2 c Cobb salad with dressing, topped with 2 oz roasted
    chicken breast
1 whole wheat dinner roll (0)
8 fl oz nonfat milk
6 oz strawberries [(4 oz)]

Snack
Yogurt and Almonds
6 oz nonfat, artificially sweetened strawberry banana yogurt
1/4 c almonds, no added salt [(1 T)]

Dinner
Carribean Chicken on Rice, Green Beans, Salad
Carribean chicken*, on 1 c brown rice (1/2 c)
1 c green beans
dinner salad: 1 1/2 c greens and mixed vegetables, topped with
    2 T oil and vinegar dressing [(1 T)]

DASH servings: 3 whole grains, 4 fruit, 4 vegetables, 4 dairy, 1
nuts, 6 oz meats

Week 4 Wednesday 2000 [1600] (1200) Calories

Breakfast
Grab & Go Toasted Pita Melt, Banana, and Juice
Grab & go toasted pita melt: 1/2 whole wheat pita bread,
    stuffed and toasted with 1 oz low sodium, low fat Swiss
    cheese [(0.6 oz)]
banana [(1/2)]
6 fl oz no added salt tomato juice [(4 fl oz)]

Lunch
Baked Potato topped with Cheesy Broccoli, Salad, Milk, and
    Plum
baked potato (1/2)
cheesy broccoli: 1 oz low sodium, low fat cheddar cheese [(0.6
    oz)] on 1/2 c broccoli
side salad: 1 c green salad and mixed vegetables, with 2 T oil
    and vinegar dressing [(1 T)]
8 fl oz nonfat milk
1 medium plum [(small)]

Snack
Apple and Peanut Butter
1 medium apple [(small)]
2 T peanut butter [(1 T)]

Dinner
Sloppy Joes, Applesauce, Peas and Carrots, Cole Slaw, and
    Yogurt Topped with Berries
*sloppy Joes** (1/3 c) on a whole wheat hamburger bun [(0)]
1/2 c applesauce, unsweetened
1 c peas and carrots
1 c Italian cole slaw [(1/2 c)]
1/2 c artificially sweetened, nonfat frozen raspberry yogurt,
    topped with 1 c mixed berries [(1/2 c)]

DASH servings: 3 whole grains, 4 fruits, 7 vegetables, 4 dairy, 1
nuts, 3 oz meats

Week 4 Thursday 2000 [1600] (1200) Calories

Breakfast
Grits, Berries, Biscuit, Juice, and Milk
1/2 c grits
1 c raspberries [((1/2 c)]
biscuit (0), topped with 2 t raspberry preserves (0)
6 fl oz pineapple juice [(4 fl oz)]
8 fl oz nonfat milk

Lunch
Pile It On! Chili Topped with Cheddar, Salad, Milk, and Apple
1 c *Pile It On! chili** (2/3 c), topped with 1 oz low sodium, low
    fat shredded cheddar cheese [(0.6 oz)]
side salad: 1 c greens and mixed vegetables, 8 grape tomatoes,
    topped with 2 T oil and vinegar dressing [(1 T)]
8 fl oz nonfat milk
1 medium apple [(small)]

Snack
Yogurt, Peach, and Peanuts
6 oz nonfat, artificially sweetened peach yogurt
peach
1/4 c peanuts, unsalted [(1 T)]

Dinner
Chicken Stir Fry on Rice, Egg Roll, and Strawberries
Marla's chicken stir fry* on 1/2 c brown rice
1 chicken egg roll [(0)]
6 oz strawberries [(4 oz)]

DASH servings: 2 whole grains, 5 fruits, 5 vegetables, 4 dairy, 1
nuts, 1 beans, 6 oz meats

Week 4 Friday 2000 [1600] (1200) Calories

Breakfast
Cereal, Blueberries, English Muffin, OJ, and Milk
1 oz shredded wheat, topped with 6 oz blueberries [(4 oz)]
1/2 mixed grain English muffin [(0)], topped with 1 t soft,
    unsalted margarine [(0)]
6 fl oz orange juice [(4 fl oz)]
8 fl oz nonfat milk

Lunch
Waldorf Stuffed Tomato, Cornbread, Snow Pea Pods, and
    Peach
Waldorf stuffed tomato: 1 c *tuna Waldorf salad** (3/4 c) in a
    tomato
1/2 cup snow pea pods
1 cup side salad with 2 T nonfat, no added salt Italian dressing
cornbread (0)
1 medium peach [(small)]

Afternoon snack
Gelatin, Cheese, and Apple
1/2 c artificially sweetened mixed fruit gelatin
1 oz Light Baby Bel™ cheese
1 medium apple [(small)]

Dinner
Lean Swiss Cheeseburger, Oven Potato Fries, Broccoli,
    Coleslaw, and Banana Split
Swiss cheeseburger: whole wheat hamburger bun [(0)], 3 oz
    broiled extra lean ground sirloin [(2 oz)], with 1 oz low fat
    Swiss cheese {(0.6 oz)], mustard and catsup
1 serving *oven potato fries** [(1/2)]
1/2 c broccoli
1 c coleslaw [(1/2 c)]
banana split: 1/2 c each nonfat, artificially sweetened chocolate
    and vanilla frozen yogurt (1/4 c each), banana (1/2) , 2 T
    chocolate syrup (1 T)

DASH servings: 4 whole grains, 5 fruit, 6 vegetables, 5 dairy,
1/2 nuts, 6 oz meats

Week 4 Saturday 2000 [1600] (1200) Calories

Breakfast
Glazed Doughnut, Banana, OJ, and Latte
glazed doughnut
banana [(1/2)]
6 fl oz fresh squeezed orange juice [(4 fl oz)]
latte: 2 fl oz espresso and 8 fl oz nonfat milk

Lunch
Soup and Half Sandwich, Milk, Cantaloupe, and Strawberries
half sandwich: 1 slice whole wheat bread, 1/2 c chicken salad
    [(1/3 c)]
3/4 c low sodium split pea soup
1 cup *Italian cole slaw** [(1/2 c)]
8 fl oz nonfat milk
6 oz cantaloupe [(4 oz)]
1 c strawberries [(1/2 c)]

Snack
Yogurt, Popcorn, and Apple
6 oz nonfat, artificially sweetened blueberry yogurt
2 c light microwave popcorn (0)
1 medium apple [(small)]

Dinner
Grilled Shrimp Kebobs, Mixed Vegetables, Salad, Milk, Peach
    Topped Frozen Yogurt
grilled shrimp kebobs: 4 oz shrimp [(3 oz)], 1/2 c pepper strips
1 c mixed cauliflower, broccoli, and carrots
dinner salad: 1 1/2 c greens and mixed vegetables, topped with
    2 T oil and vinegar dressing [(1 T)]
8 fl oz nonfat milk
1/2 c artificially sweetened, nonfat vanilla frozen yogurt,
    topped with 1 medium peach, sliced [(small)]

DASH servings: 3 whole grains, 5 fruits, 5 vegetables, 4 dairy, 1
nuts, and 7 oz meats

Week 4 Sunday 2000 [1600] (1200) Calories

Breakfast
Scrambled Eggs and Bacon, Toast, Hot Chocolate, Raspberries, and OJ
2 scrambled eggs [(1)]
2 slices bacon [(0)]
2 slices whole wheat toast [1] (0), topped with 4 t raspberry jam
    [2 t] (0)
hot chocolate: 8 fl oz nonfat milk, 1 t cocoa powder, and 2
    packages Splenda™
1 c raspberries [(1/2 c)]
6 fl oz freshly squeezed orange juice [(4 fl oz)]

Lunch
Chicken Quesadilla, Salad, and Cantaloupe
chicken quesadilla: 1 whole wheat tortilla [(1/2)], topped with
    3 oz roasted chicken breast [(2 oz)], and 1 oz low sodium,
    low fat Colby-jack cheese [(0.6 oz)]. Fold tortilla over, heat
    in toaster oven. Top with 2 T guacamole [(1 T)]
side salad: 1 c green salad with mixed vegetables, 2 T oil and
    vinegar dressing [(1 T)]
6 oz cantaloupe [(4 oz)]

Snack
Banana Strawberry Smoothie
smoothie: 8 fl oz nonfat milk, banana [(1/2)], 1 c strawberries
    [(4 oz)]

Dinner
Meat Loaf, Mashed Potatoes, Broccoli, Salad, and Frozen
    Yogurt
3 oz meat loaf
1/2 c homestyle mashed potatoes
1/2 c broccoli
dinner salad: 1 1/2 c dinner salad, 2 T oil and vinegar dressing
    [(1 T)]
1/2 c artificially sweetened, nonfat chocolate frozen yogurt

DASH servings: 3 whole grains, 5 fruits, 4 vegetables, 3+ dairy,
9 oz meats

Chapter 4 Menu Guide, DASH Meals Away from Home

Staying on track with any healthy eating plan can be a challenge when you are away from home. With a little advance planning, you can still hit the mark with the DASH diet, without being overly stressed.

If you are lucky, you get many of your meals-away-from-home at real restaurants. Most of us rely on take out or fast food restaurants too often, but we can still find food that fit into the DASH plan. Travel presents special concerns, but this is a part of real life, so we need to have DASH tips for trips, too. And special events can trip us up, if we don't think and plan before we go to the big party.

Restaurant meals

At restaurants, we have 3 key rules to help stay on track with portion size. Share. Divide and conquer. Bag it. These tips and more will help you stay the course.

1. **Split up.** If you have an agreeable spouse, partner, or friend, split entreés, large salads, and desserts.
2. **Bon appetizer.** Choose an appetizer portion instead of a main course.
3. **Basta pasta.** Basta is Italian for "Enough!"

However, most Italian restaurants serve more than enough, especially with pasta. It makes it look like you are getting good value, but you aren't getting lots of the really good stuff. To increase the DASH quotient, ask to have the sauce on steamed vegetables instead of pasta. Save the grain servings for the bread, if it is really good. If you do have the pasta, ask them to serve only a small portion of pasta, and then save the remainder to take home for several more meals.

4. **Bag it**. If you really can't stop eating when the food is in front of you, ask them to bag half (or more) before they bring it out. I had one client who found she could successfully cut her calories by putting the extra portion on a bread plate so she wouldn't keep eating, just because it was on her plate. Then she would ask to have the leftover portion wrapped.

5. **Avoid portion distortion**. Choose your portion size. Many short women who want to lose weight find that half portions are still too big to fit into their calorie allotment. You may find that one-third or a quarter of a serving is more appropriate. You decide, before you start to eat.

6. **Just desserts**. Order just one dessert for four people. This makes it easy to avoid overdoing.

7. **Side order of veggies**. Fill up on non-starchy vegetables to maximize the DASH potential of your diet, and support losing weight. Order extra vegetables.

8. **Prime isn't best**. When you are trying to follow a moderate fat diet, lower your cholesterol, or lose

weight, prime meats don't fill the bill. Prime meats have more "hidden" fat, also referred to as marbling. If you are at a restaurant with only prime meats, choose fish, or tenderloin. Tenderloin is a relatively lean cut, often called filet mignon on menus. Choose the petite filet (8 ounces) which will give you a 6-ounce portion to eat. If you have already had one serving of meat, fish, or poultry that day, only eat half of what is served at dinner. Save the rest for a meal later in the week. Half of a 6-ounce cooked serving is three ounces which is a perfect size for the DASH diet.

9. **Bread, bread, everywhere.** If bread is your downfall, tell yourself you will only have it if it is whole grain. This will cut down on your bread intake right away. If you do have bread, don't put butter on it! If bread is your weakness and you won't give it up at restaurants, ask the waiter to delay bringing the bread until your salad is served. This will eliminate the mindless bread eating that is typical of many of us at restaurants.

Fast Food Meals

Fast food makes it a little harder to keep to the DASH diet, but occasional fast food meals can fit into a flexible plan. Most fast food restaurants have salads. Add some grilled chicken and watch your salad dressing portion size, and you have a DASH-friendly meal. If you keep some portable fruit with you, such as apples, tangerines (especially

Clementine tangerines in the winter), plums, nectarines, or grapes, you will be able to add fiber and sweetness. Add a carton of skim milk and you will have added several of the key DASH foods to your day, even with fast food meals.

Travel Days

While you are on the road, it may seem difficult to stay with the DASH plan. You may not be able to make every meal DASH-friendly, but you can identify meals where you can be sure to get many of the key DASH foods, and load up when you can. Breakfast is a sure bet for fruit servings. Even McDonald's has skim milk and orange juice. Many Starbucks and other coffee house restaurants have fruit cups in addition to juice. Add a skim latte or a skim hot chocolate, and you have your nonfat dairy serving. At sit-down restaurants, order an omelette made with egg whites or egg substitute, and include peppers, onions and mushrooms. Many restaurants now offer fresh fruit instead of toast or potatoes for low carb diners at breakfast. This is a great way to keep your calories under control while you are on the road. At lunch grab a salad and grilled chicken if you are fast fooding it. If you get to eat at a real restaurant, you can have a side salad and extra vegetables. For snacks, stop and get some low fat portable cheese, a small bag of nuts, and some fruit at a grocery store. In the evening, look for restaurants where you can get good vegetable sides, great salads, and not overly fatty foods. Many of the chains have lighter options, and most local restaurants will have real vegetable sides. Restaurants that cater to low carb diners will be happy to serve extra vegetables, and may even have fresh fruit for dinner. When you go to the market to buy snacks, buy some extra fruit for your evening dessert.

Special Events

Weddings, Christenings, birthday parties, confirmations or bar/bat mitzvahs, anniversaries are all occasions that bring special challenges in staying with any eating plan. Probably the best plan is to choose a few special items that you will indulge in at the party, and try to make the rest of the day relatively on target with your DASH plan.

Restaurants

Starbucks and Other Coffee Stores

Choose a latte with 8 ounces of skim milk and 8 ounces of coffee. This gives you a full serving of milk. If you don't drink coffee, order hot chocolate made with skim milk, and skip the whipped cream. Most Starbucks locations have fruit cups with a serving of fruit. If you want a pastry, choose a bagel, but only eat half. Most bagels are 4 - 5 servings of grains. A cinnamon raisin bagel provides plenty of flavor without the extra calories and saturated fat of the cream cheese. Watch out for large juice containers which hold 2 to 2 1/2 servings. I generally recommend that people limit themselves to 1 serving of juice each day. Juice is less filling than fruit, making it easier to overdo calories.

Italian

The best part of an Italian menu are the vegetables, as antipasto and woven into most entrées. There are so many wonderful choices that will boost the DASH quotient of your meal. A variety of salads and many of the pasta toppings provide you with the opportunity to choose from many different plant-based foods. The many chicken and seafood dishes give you many choices for lean protein sources. Olive oil based dressings provide heart-healthy monounsaturated fats. Key pitfalls include cream based sauces and whole fat cheeses which are high in saturated fats, large pasta serving sizes, and overdoing bread. Many restaurants provide 4 - 8 servings of pasta on each plate. If you have had 2 - 3 pieces of bread before your meal, you can easily consume double the servings of grains that you need each day. Sometimes I recommend that people ask for a side order of vegetables, and ask to have the pasta sauce put on top of the vegetables instead of pasta. I often have my pasta sauce on green beans, but many other vegetables will also be interesting. If you have trouble limiting bread before the meal, ask the server to hold off on the bread until your salad arrives. Bread served before the food arrives often triggers mindless eating, and it doesn't fill you up enough to limit intake during the meal. Topping the bread with butter or soaking it in olive oil only adds to the calorie overload. Refined bread and pasta don't add any benefit to the DASH quotient of the meal. If you are having pizza, choose vegetable toppings, and limit yourself to a few slices of thin crust or 1 slice of thick crust pizza. Start your meal with a good sized salad to fill you up, and avoid overdoing the pizza. In Italy, typical restaurant desserts are bowls of fresh fruit rather than cannoli or tiramisu. Only 29% of Americans get even two servings of fruit each day. Choosing fresh fruit for dessert in a restaurant is a satisfying end to a wonderful meal.

Chinese

Just like Italian cuisine, Chinese foods can be rich sources of vegetables. However, they can also be full of hidden fats and loads of extra carbs. To get the maximum DASH benefit, order an extra serving of steamed vegetables. Put some of your topping on the vegetables rather than on rice. One cup of cooked rice has 200 calories. Many of us have 2 - 3 cups of rice at a Chinese restaurant which can easily put us over our allotment of grain servings and over our calorie limit. And many of the appetizers are loaded with calories. Egg rolls can have as much as 400 -600 calories **each!** Crab rangoon is loaded with cream cheese; fried pot stickers are equally high in calories. Choose appetizers which have not been fried to minimize your calorie intake. Steamed appetizers or soup would be a better choice.

American Casual

Many chain restaurants are competing based on providing more value for the money. This usually takes the form of large portions. The first trick is to cut down the portion size. Share with a friend or ask the server to bag half before they bring out the dish. Then decide if it is still too large. Identify how much you want to eat from the very start, and get it off your plate. Use your bread plate to hold the part that you don't want to eat (at that meal). If it stays on your plate, you will probably eat it. If you like hearty portions, order extra vegetables (without butter, cheese, or too much oil) and fill up on non-starchy vegetables. Watch out for sautéed or grilled vegetables. These are typically oil-laden and bursting with extra calories. (Grilled vegetables tend to soak up cooking oil like a sponge, unlike grilled meats, which tend to lose fat in the cooking process.)

Restaurant food often has extra-rich flavors due to extra toppings, especially those with large amounts of cheese. While cheese is a great calcium-rich DASH food, large amounts of full-fat cheese pile on extra calories and loads of saturated fats. These cheeses can come in salads, on pizza (and sometimes stuffed in the crust), in pasta toppings, sandwiches, and on top of meat or chicken. Leave the cheese off the salad, and limit portion sizes of the other cheese-rich foods.

Fast Food

The fast food industry has been under attack for

causing obesity in children and adults. Fast food has become a mainstay of American culture in our overscheduled lives. Making smart choices at fast food restaurants can be challenging, but it can be done.

Most restaurants have salads. Choose grilled chicken instead of crispy, and limit your serving size on dressing if you choose a full-fat dressing. If you want a sandwich choose the smallest burger or a grilled chicken sandwich. If you need to limit carbs at this meal, remove half the bun. If the chain has a sandwich with lettuce and tomatoes this can be a good choice, but it may be only available on larger sandwiches which will lead to more calories. If you absolutely have to add fries to your meal, order the small serving and throw out half before you start eating (or split it with a friend or your kids). Potatoes are rich in potassium, but you don't need the extra calories from the fat. Some chicken sandwiches have more calories and fat than others, so check the on-line nutrient listings via our links at dashdiet.org. Add a carton of skim milk to increase the DASH benefits of your meal. Some franchises are now offering fresh fruits, so take advantage if this is available.

Since portion size is so critical, you really want to avoid the impulse to "super size" or "biggie size" your meals. At fast food restaurants, we are unlikely to save part of the meal for another day; we tend to eat everything that we purchase. Reframe your idea on what makes for good value in a meal.

Traditionally we consider a meal to be a good value if we get a lot for our money. However, for many of us, this means that we overeat and get fatter from foods that add little nutritional value. A better concept for the DASH diet is to consider good value to be a meal that is rich in fruits, vegetables, low-fat dairy, and lean meats, fish, or poultry. A good value DASH meal is not heavy in fats or refined carbohydrates. Your first priority is to choose foods that improve your health, not foods that expand your waistline.

Sandwich restaurants seem like a good choice, since the foods are not fried (except for the extra-large-sized chips sold with the meals). However, they are often unbalanced in terms of the ratio of refined grains to protein. For example a 6" turkey sub from Subway™ contains 3 servings of bread and 1 ounce (⅓ serving) of turkey. Yes, you can add vegetables, which is great, but you are getting lots of carbs and too little protein. This is a meal that may leave you hungry an hour or two later. A better choice is to order the roasted chicken, which comes in a 2 ounce serving, and to lose the top part of the bread. Surprisingly, there is no fiber advantage if you compare their "whole wheat" versus the other breads. The key to keeping calories under control in the sandwich shops is to watch out for the bread serving size. You also want to avoid eating an entire large bag of chips. These are often the Big Grab™ size, which holds 2 1/2 ounces. Even when you choose baked chips, you are getting lots of calories.

Try to limit yourself to a small handful, and toss the rest. Remember, it is more wasteful to consume extra calories and increase your health risk, than to throw away extra food.

Sauces, dressings, and toppings are another source of extra calories. Mustard, ketchup, veggies, salsa, and low fat mayonnaise are good toppings. You want to limit regular mayonnaise, oil, sour cream, and large servings of regular salad dressing. For example, at salad bars, many people use 1/2 cup of salad dressing or more. Regular dressing has a whopping 500 calories per 1/2 cup. You can avoid overdoing, by avoiding thick dressings, such as Thousand Island. A better choice would be "slippery" dressings such as Italian, which covers a lot of salad without too much dressing. Any excess ends up on our plate. The mayonnaise that tops many sandwiches is 3/4 ounce, which adds 160 calories to the sandwich. Request no mayonnaise, or ask them to just use a little. A baked potato topped with broccoli and cheese has 55% additional calories than a plain baked potato. Since 1/2 cup of broccoli only has 25 calories, clearly the extra calories come from the ful-fat cheese. Toppings can take a meal that has relatively moderate calories and push it over the top, so limit high fat extras.

On the Job

Some workplaces really make it difficult to stay with a healthy eating plan. Too little time and limited choices make for conditions which probably led to overweight and hypertension in the first place. However, you can choose to take charge of your health, and eat great, even at work.

Some companies have cafeterias, which can be great for getting more variety. Most cafeterias have some kind of salad bar. Stock up on non-mayonnaise-based veggies and fruits. Get a serving of cooked vegetables. Add skim milk or light yogurts. If your cafeteria is lacking in some of your favorites, talk to the manager and make some recommendations. The key DASH foods are healthy choices, also great for people who are watching their weight. With so many people trying to watch their weight and eat more healthfully, even if you have to take the lead in adding to the menu offerings, you won't be the only one who will take advantage of the new choices.

If you have access to a refrigerator, stock it up with yogurt, fruit, raw veggies, light cheeses, milk chugs. Or bring a few of these in an insulated bag with an frozen cooling bag.

Meetings and people who bring in treats can present challenging obstacles to your DASH plan, especially if you are trying to lose weight. If you bring healthy shacks to work and avoid getting overly hungry, you won't be as tempted by office treats or birthday cakes. Hunger leads to diminished resolve when it comes to avoiding empty calorie treats. In the morning, if you have some light yogurt or fresh fruit, you won't be tempted to eat several doughnuts, or an entire bagel slathered with cream cheese. Ask meeting planners to include some fresh fruit or raw veggies. Or you could be the one to bring in a fruit tray or a bowl of apples rather than a box of doughnuts. If your boss rewards extra work with a pizza party, try to stick with just one slice, have a piece of fruit, and then have a smaller dinner, with an emphasis on low calorie veggies. If you see a candy jar that seems to be calling to you, get back to your desk and have a piece of light cheese and some fruit or some yogurt and nuts. If your choice is between having nothing versus indulging in diet-busting foods, chances are that you will give in to temptation. Keep healthy snack foods on hand.

The key to watching your weight and following the DASH guidelines is to plan ahead. Think about what you need for the whole day. How will your meals away from home fit into your DASH plan? Restaurant meals are not a surprise, they are typical for most of us. When you know you will be eating away from home, plan ahead, and think about your choices. Do you need some vegetables and low fat dairy at this meal? Envision what you will order, before you look at the menu or stand in line at a fast food place. Then you will be less likely to choose a tempting, but empty calorie meal, and you will meet your DASH objectives every day.

Chapter 4 DASHboard

Surviving restaurant meals.
1. Plan what you will choose, before you go.
2. Manage portion sizes by sharing, choosing smaller servings, or taking half (or more) home. Many entrees and desserts can easily serve 3 - 4 people
3. Choose lean meats, poultry, or fish.
4. Limit bread to whole grains or hold off on the bread basket until your salad arrives.
5. Choose salads at fast food outlets, and skim milk as a side. Carry portable fruit to round out the meal.
6. On the road, buy fruits, low fat individually packaged cheese, and unsalted nuts to complement restaurant meals.

Tracking my Personal DASH Diet Action Plan:

3 specific changes I will make at restaurants or at work:

_____
_____
_____

Chapter 5 DASH Your Way to Weight Loss

The DASH diet makes it easy to lose weight. A healthy diet, one that is based on fruits, vegetables, and other key DASH foods, will help you have satisfying meals, without overeating. And new research shows that including calcium-rich dairy foods in your diet can have special benefits for weight loss. So, DASH provides the perfect foundation for a weight loss plan.

Losing weight is recommended as one of the key lifestyle changes to help manage high blood pressure. Even greater advantages can be expected when weight loss is combined with the DASH diet plan. In this chapter, you will learn how to identify your healthy weight, calculate the calories you need to reach that goal, and learn specific weight loss strategies.

Research has shown that foods in the DASH diet can support weight loss. With a diet rich in fruits and vegetables, you can fill up without overdoing calories. Lean meat, fish and poultry provide satiating protein with fewer calories than higher fat meats. For example, 8 ounces of boiled shrimp has the same calories as 3 ounces of corned beef, while providing more satisfaction. Low-fat dairy foods have much fewer calories than the higher fat versions they replace. And research suggests that diets rich in dairy calcium promote weight loss, especially with reducing extra fat around your waist.

Being overweight is a primary risk factor for developing high blood pressure. For children and teens, extra weight is even riskier. Parents with high blood pressure, who adopt the DASH diet, help their kids significantly by providing the right foods and avoiding calorie-laden meals. Children learn eating patterns by observing their parents. As a parent, you can model healthy behavior, and help your kids avoid a lifetime regimen of blood pressure medication. Knowing that your actions are important for the whole family can provide strong motivation to follow through on your own diet and lifestyle changes.

What is a healthy weight?

There are many ways to evaluate whether your weight is healthy for you. The Metropolitan Life Weight Tables were used for many years to identify healthy weights. Recently BMI (body mass index, which show the relation of weight to height) has become an important tool for assessing healthy weight. Body fat percentage is another indicator of fitness (or fatness). And some health professionals believe that a healthy weight is the weight at which you do not have health issues, or at least none related to your weight.

In 1998, the National Institutes of Health issued new guidelines for healthy weight, based on BMI. They were developed to provide information on the ratio of weight to height that was associated with lower risk of disease. BMI is based on a formula of weight in kilograms divided by height in meters, squared. The following table lets you find your BMI (without a calculator) and shows you where your weight falls in terms of health risks. It is important to realize that not everyone who is in the elevated risk category is truly at higher risk for disease. The BMI tables reflect generalized risk for large numbers of people, but not for each individual. For example, a sedentary person who is at a healthy weight might have higher risk for disease than someone who is overweight, but physically fit. And a football player would look overweight by the BMI tables, although he is probably not overfat.

A BMI of less than 19 is considered to be underweight, 19 - 25 is a healthy weight, 26 - 30 is overweight, 31 - 39 is obese, and BMI greater than 40 is considered to be very obese.

Fitness (or fatness) can be measured by looking at body fat percentage. Body fat percentage can be evaluated in several ways. In a research setting (and some physician offices), body fat can be measured by DEXA (dual emission X-ray analysis) which can be done on the same equipment that is used for performing bone mineral density scans. This is considered to be the best procedure. Inexpensive bio-electrical impedance analysis (BIA) devices

BMI (Body Mass Index)

Find your height in inches at left, follow across to your weight; the top of the column indicates your BMI.

Height (inches) \ BMI	18	19	20	21	22	23	24	25	26	27	28	29	30	31	32	33	34	35	36	37	38	39	40
58	86	91	96	100	105	110	115	120	124	129	134	139	144	148	153	158	163	167	172	177	182	187	191
59	89	94	99	104	109	114	119	124	129	134	139	144	149	153	158	163	168	173	178	183	188	193	198
60	92	97	102	108	113	118	123	128	133	138	143	148	154	159	164	169	174	179	184	189	195	200	205
61	95	101	106	111	116	122	127	132	137	143	148	153	159	164	169	175	180	185	191	196	201	206	212
62	98	104	109	115	120	126	131	137	142	147	153	158	164	169	175	180	186	192	197	202	208	213	219
63	102	107	113	119	124	130	135	141	147	152	158	164	169	175	180	186	192	198	203	209	215	220	226
64	105	110	116	122	128	134	140	146	151	157	163	169	174	180	186	192	198	204	210	216	221	227	233
65	108	114	120	126	132	138	144	150	156	162	168	174	180	186	192	198	204	210	216	222	228	234	240
66	112	118	124	130	136	142	148	155	161	167	173	179	186	192	198	204	211	217	223	229	235	242	248
67	115	121	127	134	140	146	153	160	166	172	178	185	191	198	204	211	217	223	230	236	243	249	255
68	118	125	131	138	144	151	158	164	171	177	184	190	197	203	210	216	223	230	237	243	250	256	263
69	122	128	135	142	149	155	162	169	176	182	189	196	203	209	216	223	230	237	243	249	256	264	271
70	125	132	139	146	153	160	167	174	181	188	195	202	209	216	222	229	236	243	250	257	264	272	279
71	129	136	143	151	158	165	172	179	186	194	201	208	215	222	229	237	244	251	258	265	272	280	287
72	133	140	147	155	162	170	177	184	192	199	206	214	221	229	236	243	251	258	265	273	280	288	295
73	136	144	152	159	167	174	182	189	197	205	212	220	227	235	243	250	258	265	273	280	288	296	303
74	140	148	156	164	172	180	187	195	203	210	218	226	234	241	249	257	265	273	280	288	296	304	312
75	144	152	160	168	176	184	192	200	208	216	224	232	240	248	256	264	272	280	288	296	304	312	320
76	148	156	164	173	181	189	197	205	214	222	230	238	246	255	263	271	279	288	296	304	312	320	329
77	152	160	169	177	186	194	202	211	219	228	236	245	253	261	270	278	287	295	304	312	320	329	337
78	156	164	173	182	190	199	208	216	225	234	242	251	260	268	277	286	294	303	312	320	329	337	346
79	160	169	178	186	195	204	213	222	231	240	249	257	266	275	284	293	302	311	320	328	337	346	355
80	164	173	182	191	200	209	218	228	237	246	255	264	273	282	291	300	309	319	328	337	346	355	364
81	168	177	187	196	205	215	224	233	243	252	261	271	280	289	299	308	317	327	336	345	355	364	373
82	172	182	191	201	210	220	230	239	249	258	268	277	287	296	306	316	325	335	344	354	363	373	383

for home use can provide useful information and are available in tools such as a hand-held device that is gripped like a steering wheel, or some home scales. Underwater weighing is another way to measure body fat and is performed at some health clubs. Healthy body fat percentages are shown in the table below. The average American man has a 24.5% body fat percentage, and the average woman has 33% body fat.

Suggested percent body fat standards for adults.		
	Men	Women
Lean	<8	<15
Optimal health	8-15	15-22
Slightly overweight	16-20	23-26
Fat	21-24	27-32
Obese or overfat	25+	32+

Waist size is another way healthy weight indicator. Waist circumference is used to evaluate whether you might be at increased risk for certain diseases. You may be familiar with the concept of apple versus pear physiques. People who carry most of their extra fat in their waist (apple-shaped) are at higher risk for heart disease, type 2 diabetes, and certain types of cancer, compared to people who carry extra weight in their hips (pear-shaped). If waist circumference is larger than 35 inches for women or 40 inches for men, it is probably a good idea to lose weight and increase physical activity.

Another concept of a healthy weight holds that it is possible to be healthy and yet be heavier than normal. If you have high blood pressure and you are overweight, then this would not apply to you. You will most likely benefit from some weight reduction. As with everything, we need to use our judgement when deciding on a healthy weight for any specific person.

Deciding on your healthy weight goal

You can decide what your target weight will be. It will probably be somewhere in the healthy BMI zone. If you have a long way to go, you might set a short term goal to lose about 10% of your total weight. Many research studies have shown that people can significantly improve their health if they lose 7 to 10% of their weight.

Your starting weight   _____

Starting date   _____

Your target weight   _____

Date expected to reach   _____

Now that you have selected a target weight, you need to decide how much you can safely lose each week. Typically, nutrition professionals think that women can lose about 1- 2 pounds per week and men can lose 2 - 4 pounds per week (perhaps more at the beginning, for people who have more to lose). Your goal is to lose fat and maintain muscle. If you lose weight too fast, you may lose muscle and slow down your metabolism. The DASH diet plan which has plenty of low fat protein foods, calcium-rich dairy, high fiber fruits, vegetables, and whole grains will support healthy weight loss.

What are your calorie needs?
To lose 1 pound per week, you will need to reduce your calorie intake by 500 calories per day. In order to evaluate your diet plan, you need to estimate your daily calorie needs. We have many sophisticated formulas that will estimate your calorie needs. There are even machines that can directly evaluate your metabolic rate. For most people, it is practical to estimate needs based on the following guidelines.

Estimating calorie needs for weight maintenance.		
Activity level	Calories per pound body weight	Calories per kilogram body weight
Sedentary	13.5	30
Moderate	16	35
Heavy	18	40

Multiply your weight by the calories per pound, and you will have the amount of calories that you need to maintain your weight. Then subtract 500 calories in order to lose 1 pound per week (or 1000 if you want to lose 2 pounds per week).

Current weight   _____

Calories per pound   X   _____

Calories to maintain   =   _____

Minus calories to lose   -   _____

Target calories   =   _____

Adding exercise to your weight loss program will help you have a more generous calorie allotment, and it will also help lower your blood pressure and improve cardiovascular fitness. See chapter 6 for more information on the payoff from exercise and specific recommendations to help you meet your goals.

Your target calories will be used to determine the number of servings you need from the DASH diet. You should not go lower than 1200 calories per day. Below this intake, it will be difficult to get enough of the key DASH foods, and the diet will probably not provide a healthy balance of foods. Your objective is to improve your health, and to have a plan that is sustainable for the long run. Moderate weight loss through healthy eating and exercise will reduce your blood pressure and reduce other health risks, such as cancer and heart disease.

Weight loss strategies

There are several important strategies that will help you lose weight. One is to be sure that you are not overeating. This seems obvious, but portion sizes are increasing at restaurants, in convenience foods, packaged foods, and even in recipes. The next section will key you in on how to avoid "portion distortion." Extra calories can also sneak in through foods that are fattening. This seems obvious, but there are many foods that are "calorie-dense," which means that extra calories are packed into a normal-sized serving. For example, one national steakhouse chain provides croissants with their dinner salad. The croissants have 400 or more calories each, compared with 80 calories for a slice of bread. Then the salad is topped with over 1 ounce of full-fat cheese and a generous serving of bacon. The salad course alone will contribute at least 1000 calories. This makes it a little easier to see how Americans are getting fatter without feeling like they are doing anything different.

When you are eating at home, food labels will help you get a handle on how much you eat. Many of the foods that everyone thinks are quite healthful may provide relatively empty calories, without being filling, and can lead to eating more calories than you realize. Chapter 11 provides all the information to help you decipher the Nutrition Facts food labels.

Avoid Portion Distortion

Buy a digital scale - no not for you, for the food! Getting a handle on portion size is the first step in weight loss. If you measure and weigh your foods at home, you will be better able to estimate portion sizes in restaurants.

At home many of us underestimate how much we eat, in several ways. Cereal provides a good example, since it is very easy to underestimate portion size. Many cereal bowls hold 2 or more cups of cereal. And many cereals are quite calorie-dense. It is especially important to read the labels of cereals. A DASH-serving is 1 ounce by weight. Some of the high fiber cereals are the worst in terms of packing in a lot of calories in a small serving size. For example Grape Nuts™ have 105 calories for a 1-ounce serving which measures only 1/4 cup. A full cup of Grape Nuts would give 420 calories. Bran Buds ™ have 70 calories for a 1-ounce serving, measuring ⅓ cup. If you have 1 cup for breakfast, you are consuming 210 calories, without the milk. If you prefer more volume, you might want to choose flaked or puffed cereals, such as Grape Nut Flakes ™ where a 1-ounce serving is ⅞ cup, for 105 calories. Oatmeal is another cereal source of "portion distortion." A DASH-serving of cooked oatmeal is 1/2 cup. Pre-packaged instant oatmeal may contain 2 servings of oatmeal. You can increase the volume of smaller-sized cereal servings by topping them with berries or other sliced fruit. This improves the DASH score of your breakfast, and allows you to sweeten without adding sugar and extra calories.

When you are measuring foods remember that the servings sizes refer to cooked portions for foods that are normally cooked. The following table will show you the DASH serving sizes. These are not always the same as the servings on food labels or the diabetic exchanges. A more detailed list is found on our web site at http://dashdiet.org/servingsizes.htm.

Another source of serving size error is confusing weight measures with volume measures. In this book we will call weight measures ounces, and volume measures will be called fluid ounces. For example 1 ounce (by weight) of cereal might be 1/4 cup (2 fluid ounces) or 1 cup (8 fluid ounces). When you weigh the foods with a digital scale, you avoid this problem.

DASH diet serving sizes.	
Grains, starches	1 slice of bread 1/2 English muffin or bun 1/4 bagel 1 ounce dry cereal 1/2 cup cooked cereal, pasta, corn ⅓ cup rice
Fruits	6 ounces by weight 6 ounces of juice 1 medium piece of fruit 1/2 cup canned, frozen 1/4 cup dried fruit
Vegetables	1/2 cup cooked or raw vegetables 1 cup leafy raw vegetables 6 ounces vegetable juice
Dairy	8 fluid ounces (1 cup) milk, yogurt 1 1/2 ounces of cheese 2 cups cottage cheese (note: higher calories than other dairy servings)
Meats, fish, poultry	2 1/2 - 3 1/2 ounces, cooked
Eggs	1 egg 2 egg whites 1 fluid ounce egg-substitute
Beans	1/4 cup cooked beans, lentils, or peas
Nuts	1/4 cup or 1 ounces nuts 2 Tbsp or 1 ounce seeds 2 Tbsp peanut butter
Fats and oils	1 tsp soft margarine 1 Tbsp low fat mayonnaise 2 Tbsp light salad dressing 1 tsp vegetable oil

Avoid Calorie Creep

Many of us enjoy restaurants that provide large portions. We feel like we are getting good value for our money. However, most of us tend to eat more when we are served large portions. Even when you know you are full, it is easy to add several extra bites of dinner, while waiting for others to finish. Here are several tricks for avoiding overeating in restaurants.

1. Choose the portion that you would like to eat, and bag the rest. Some people find it easier to ask the restaurant to wrap half of the meal before it comes to the table. Others put the excess food on the bread plate before eating. If you don't want to call attention to your method, mentally choose the portion that you want, and plan to stop when you have reached it.

2. Split entrées with your spouse or a friend. Surprisingly, most of these "half-portions" look like normal serving sizes. See how we have been tricked?

3. Split larger salads.

4. Choose an appetizer portion for your main course.

5. Watch out for pasta meals. Very often the serving size is 4 - 6 times your target serving size. Eating half would still put you way over your calorie goals.

6. Ask restaurants to leave off cheese and bacon toppings on salads, or ask for it on the side, and only have a tiny portion.

7. Choose "slippery" dressings like vinaigrette or oil and vinegar. Less salad dressing is needed

and much of it ends up on the plate.

8. Ask the waiter not to bring the bread until the salad course arrives. It is easy to mindlessly overeat bread when you are sitting in a restaurant filled with the smell of good food.

9. Spend more time paying attention to the dinner conversation and looking at your dinner companions rather than at the food. You may find that you forget to eat as much.

10. Split desserts. Some national chains have dessert portions sizes that can easily feed 6 and still leave everyone satisfied.

Lose Fat, Not Muscle

Muscle is our energy-burning powerhouse. Fat just goes along for the ride, storing up extra calories. As you lose weight, you want to maintain or increase your muscle tissue, and you would like to lose extra fat. Fast weight loss often causes people to lose muscle, which slows their metabolism. This usually leads to even quicker weight regain. A balanced eating plan with adequate protein and plenty of dairy calcium will help you reach your goals and maintain your weight, fitness, and health goals. If you want to maintain muscle, clearly exercise needs to be a part of your healthy weight loss plan. Chapter 6 will help you with exercise plans that boost your muscle power and burn off fat.

Plan, plan, plan

Planning to succeed really does pay off.

1. Make sure you keep all the right foods on hand. Stock up on the key DASH foods when you

grocery shop. Buy more than you think you need.

2. Take key DASH diet foods (fruit, raw veggies, dairy) for your lunches and snacks to work. Stock your mini fridge at the office, or bring an insulated bag with all the right foods.
3. Plan to include key DASH foods in your afternoon snacks.
4. Hit the salad bar for cut up fresh veggies and fruit.
5. Buy low fat cheese that is individually packaged. Examples are Kraft 2% Singles, light string cheese, light Mini Baby Bel cheese, The Laughing Cow light spreadable cheese.
6. Buy lots of nonfat, artificially sweetened yogurt in many flavors.
7. Buy frozen vegetables in mass quantities. (I often buy 5 - 10 packages at a time, for a 2-person household.)
8. Do not skip meals or snacks. Satisfy your hunger while it is manageable.
9. Plan what you will eat for each meal and snack, each day.
10. Plan what you will eat **before** you go to a restaurant.
11. Remember your goal. Then plan to succeed.

Plan to have healthy choices available. If you consistently have trouble getting enough servings of some of the DASH food groups, plan to add them to your snacks. Yogurt, light string cheese, and even a carton of skim milk all are satisfying dairy foods for a snack. Add some fresh fruit or a handful of nuts.

Chomp on some cut up vegetables. Many people fall off track in mid to late afternoon, and hit the vending machines for candy, chips, or pop. Plan to have an afternoon snack, and make sure you have healthy choices.

Pay special attention to the dairy foods. Try to include 3 - 4 servings each day. Dairy foods have been shown to help you become more lean, which is the goal of weight loss. Make sure that the overwhelming majority of your dairy is low fat or non-fat.

When you are going out to dinner, think about what you will order. Check out Appendix A for the list of lean meats. Plan on adding some vegetables. Even if you are just going out for a burger, plan to have a salad, and side order of steamed vegetables. (And plan to only have half the burger, since most restaurant portions tend to be large.) Plan to have an extra vegetable-rich dish at Chinese restaurants or ask for a side dish of steamed vegetables. Limit your rice to one large spoonful, and use the steamed vegetables as the base for the rest of your meal. If you are going to splurge at night and have some less than healthy foods, stick to fruits, vegetables, and non-fat dairy at lunch, and try to limit the dinner portion size. Skip the bread at dinner, and taste someone else's appetizer (without ordering one for yourself). A shared dessert will help keep the calories under control.

Focus on filling up with the DASH diet foods, and weight loss will be much simpler than you think.

Chapter 5 DASHboard

1. Use the BMI table to find your healthy weight range.
2. Calculate your calorie needs.
3. Take special care to avoid "portion distortion."
4. Lose fat - not muscle. Add exercise to your routine, and get adequate protein in your diet.
5. Stock up and fill up on lower calorie DASH diet foods.

Tracking my Personal DASH Diet Action Plan:

My current weight _____

My goal weight _____

My target calories _____

My 2 biggest calorie challenges are _____

_____

_____

I will avoid these by _____

_____

_____

What will keep me motivated?_____

_____

_____

Chapter 6 Exercise Your Right to Lower Blood Pressure

Exercise is an important tool to help you to lower your blood pressure. It also can improve cardiovascular health, reducing the risk of heart disease. It can also reduce your risk of certain types of cancer. Beyond all the health benefits, exercise makes you feel younger. Most of my clients find that their energy level is much higher within the first month of starting an exercise program. There is energy in their step, and they feel great. Exercise also helps improve mood, may relieve some symptoms of depression, and is a great stress-reliever.

So why aren't we all already exercising? Many of us have very sedentary jobs, and we balance this with more inactivity at home. Running around happens in the car, not by foot.

What are the special advantages of exercise for people with hypertension? Improving cardiovascular fitness can provide significant reductions in both systolic and diastolic blood pressure. Other heart disease risk factors can be reduced, such as obesity, the ratio of bad and good cholesterol, and the risk of developing type 2 diabetes. All of these heart disease risk factors are more common in people with hypertension than they are in the general population. People who are more fit have lower death rates than unfit people with normal blood pressure. Exercise has the potential to have striking benefits for improving long term health for people with high blood pressure.

How much exercise do I need?

People who have sedentary jobs may find that they need to exercise one-hour each day just to keep even with what people with more active jobs do in their normal day. This doesn't seem fair. However, many people with sedentary jobs find that their total steps each day, as measured by a pedometer, are very low.

Take the pedometer challenge. Buy a pedometer (not the least expensive, it may not work properly or it may die quickly). Wear the pedometer all day. The average American takes 5,000 steps per day. If your number is much lower than this, you may need to schedule longer exercise sessions. The goal is to take at least 10,000 steps each day. The pedometer is an excellent tool to provide instant feed back on your activity level. And it helps you track your progress in adding small changes into your routine.

These small changes can have a big payoff in increasing your overall activity level and burning more calories. Look at the following easy-to-make changes that will increase your activity without needing extra time or special equipment.

1. Park your car farther away in the parking lot. In addition to saving your doors from dings, you add extra steps to your day, and save time by not driving around in circles looking for a closer space. Do this at the mall, the grocery store, at work. If you drive to work in a large city, find a parking garage that is farther from your office.

2. Take the train, bus, or subway to work. Each of these public transportation choices will provide you with extra walking time every weekday. They also can reduce stress, since you don't have to fight traffic to get to work. Read the paper, prepare for that presentation you have to make. Riding public transportation makes useful, "found time."

3. Climb the stairs. Walk up one floor and down two floors. As you become more fit, walk up two or more floors, and down at least 5 flights. At the office, use the bathrooms on a higher floor, and walk up and down. At home, don't make piles at the bottom of the stairs going up or at the top of stairs going down. Take things upstairs (or downstairs) each time you find something that needs to be in another spot.

4. When you get to work, do some extra walking. Walk around the block once before going in. Walk to the opposite side of the building and

then walk to your workplace.

5. Walk at lunch. Spend at least 15 minutes walking at lunch. It will rev you up for the rest of the day, and banish the mid-day droops.

Caution: Before starting an exercise program, any individual with hypertension should consult with his or her physician regarding their fitness for an exercise program, and any restrictions. Many universities with exercise physiology programs have the capability of doing extensive evaluations of fitness levels, and designing exercise programs that are appropriate to improve overall fitness.

Exercise guidelines

The American College of Sports Medicine (ACSM) is the leading group of practitioners who research and make recommendations on exercise guidelines for Americans. All of the recommendations in this section are based on position papers of the ACSM.

Exercise guidelines are generally based on 3 principles: frequency, intensity, and duration. Your routine should be designed to improve cardiovascular fitness, muscle strength, flexibility, and balance, all of which contribute to a better quality of life.

Exercise benefits

Exercise improves our quality of life. You will see improvements in:

- balance
- strengthened bones
- reduced body fat
- increased muscle mass
- improved digestive function
- metabolism boost
- lower mortality rate
- ease of performing daily activities
- improved lipid profiles (lower cholesterol, LDL, and triglycerides, and higher HDL)
- improved cardiac efficiency
- lower resting heart rate
- lower blood pressure
- increased joint mobility
- increased self-confidence
- reduced feeling of pain
- prevention of or decrease in symptoms of depression
- improved ability to manage stress
- increased intellectual function

Exercise recommendations

It is recommended that adults adopt a well-balanced exercise regimen that includes aerobic activity, strength-building exercise, stretching and balance exercises.

Resistance exercise.

This is also known as strength training, and helps to boost metabolism, making it easier to reach and maintain a healthy weight. You can participate in strength training at a gym or health club, your local senior center, or at home. At the end of this chapter is a listing of books and other resources to help you design your strength training program.

People with high blood pressure may be more likely to develop overly high blood pressure while doing resistance (strength) exercises. If you are planning an intensive strength training regimen, check with your physician regarding his or her recommendations for maximum diastolic blood pressure after exercise. Check your blood pressure immediately after each resistance exercise. If your diastolic blood pressure is higher than recommended, you may need to exercise with less resistance (less weight). You should also inform your physician about your response to the exercise.

Endurance exercise

This is also known as aerobic activity. It can lower systolic and diastolic blood pressure about 10 points. You don't have to overdo it, since moderate intensity exercise may be more beneficial than high intensity

Judging Aerobic Exercise Intensity
Moderate intensity - you can talk with ease
High intensity - it is difficult to talk, or say more than a few words at a time

exercise. And it is helpful to start slowly and then increase intensity as your endurance improves. Aerobic activity includes walking, running, biking, dancing, hiking, and more. It will improve your cardiovascular fitness and help to reduce body fat, especially around your middle.

Your goal is to try to include at least 30 minutes of aerobic activity most days of the week. If you find it difficult to find 30 minutes, then break it into three 10-minute sessions.

Flexibility exercise

This is also known as stretching. Stretching has the ability to provide immediate benefits in your well-being. It can reduce the pain of arthritis, help prevent and recover from injuries, and can help in preventing falls. Joints get nourishment from the surrounding fluid when they are flexed and relaxed, so stretching may help you feel less stiff and achy – and younger.

Balance exercise

Preventing falls is a major objective as we get older. Many types of exercise can improve balance, such as yoga, T'ai Chi, and other simple exercises. Some books and other resources with simple balance exercises are shown at the end of this chapter.

Basic Exercise Guidelines

A basic exercise routine includes each of the exercise types, aerobic, resistance, flexibility, and balance each week. Try to do aerobic, stretching and balance exercise most days, and add some kind of resistance exercise 2 - 3 days per week (with at least one day in between).

Plan to do some exercise each day. If you plan to exercise 7 days a week, you are more likely to exercise at least 5 days. If you plan to exercise 5 days a week, schedule conflicts are likely to reduce it to only 3 days.

Plan to exercise 60 minutes each day if you are trying to lose weight. Weight maintainers may be able to get by with only 30 minutes per day.

Stay hydrated while you exercise. Consume 8 - 16 ounces before aerobic exercise, and 4 - 8 ounces every 15 - 20 minutes during exercise. After exercise include both carbs and protein in your snack or meal.

Exercise - How to Fit It In, How to Stick with It

Since many of us do not exercise enough or at all, it requires concerted effort to make exercise a part of your daily routine. You need to choose exercise that you will enjoy and then make it easy for you to participate.

For many people, exercise is more likely to fit into their schedule if they can do it at home. This saves a lot of time. You don't have to drive anywhere, you don't have to bring a bag with all your clothes (and probably forget some critical item). Whether you exercise first thing in the morning or in the evening, if you exercise at home, it is more likely to get done. Home equipment can include treadmill, exercise bike, elliptical trainer, or weight machines. Exercising at home can be as simple as running in your neighborhood or in a local park or dancing to music at home. Jump ropes, mini-tramps, roller blades, and free weights are all very inexpensive home exercise equipment.

It is important to choose a type of exercise that you enjoy. You may think that you don't enjoy any exercise. If so, you will benefit from finding something to do while you exercise to make it more enjoyable. Many people enjoy listening to music, watching a movie, listening to a book on tape, watching the news or a favorite show. In my experience (and that of many of my clients), morning news shows tend have very short segments. This causes you to focus more on the time, and seems to make the exercise seem to drag on and on. National Public Radio may be a better choice for the news to accompany your exercise, since its segments run 10 minutes. If you don't like to exercise, you need something to provide entertaining distraction during your entire exercise routine.

Personality is also important for making your exercise choices. Some people like to exercise in groups, and find that motivating. Health clubs, YMCAs, senior centers, and park districts all provide great exercise opportunities for people who like group exercise. Find a friend who likes to do the same thing as you do, if you respond to peer pressure. Shop carefully for an exercise club where you feel comfortable. Being at a club with lots of people in spandex could inspire you to exercise harder, or it could make you reluctant to even show up. Some overweight women may feel more comfortable at female-only clubs. Many people like team sports, such as softball or basketball, or competitive individual sports such as golf or tennis.

If you find it hard to self-motivate, you may want to set up session with a personal trainer, either at a club or at home.

Exercise can improve your balance, make you stronger, or improve your stamina. Exercise will help you feel younger. The point is to find something that suits your time needs, personality, fitness level, and body comfort level. And do it!

Following are many great ideas for adding active time to your life.

walking	yoga	circuit training
jogging	t'ai-chi	weight
running	karate	training
long-distance	rowing	body building
running	canoeing	Pilates
triathalons	kayaking	exercise ball
inline skating	swimming	free weights
frisbee	synchronized	aerobics
stretching	swimming	aerobic dance
gardening	ice skating	jazz dance

square dancing	cycling	calisthenics
belly dancing	curling skiing	stationary
ballroom	mountaineering	bike
dancing	jumping rope	run on
folk dancing	basketball	treadmill
ballet	softball	mini-trampoline
mountain	racquetball	
biking	handball	
hiking	tennis	
walking/hiking	golf	
clubs	hockey	

Getting Started

How do you get on track with your exercise routine? You may need to get exercise clothes and shoes, some home exercise equipment, and find a gym or other place to exercise. Set the stage for success by breaking down the barriers.

Make sure you get good shoes for the type of activity you plan to do. Your gym shoes should provide good support for your foot and walking style. If you find it difficult to bend over and tie your shoes, try to find slip on gym shoes.

If it fits into your budget and into your living space, invest in good exercise equipment. A home treadmill, elliptical trainer, cross-country ski machine, or other aerobic equipment will make it easy to exercise in all weather conditions. Free weights allow you to become stronger. Exercise balls, bands, ramps and more can increase fun and decrease boredom. EBay or second hand stores can be an inexpensive source of home equipment.

Burn a CD with your favorite tunes for your walking or running program. Get a book on tape from your local library. Get a portable radio, CD or MP3 player, or cassette deck. Put a TV and a DVD player in front of your treadmill, or set up a boom box with a remote control to pump up the volume as you exercise harder. Find something to make the time you spend exercising more enjoyable.

Make your plan for your exercise routine. When will you exercise? Where will it happen. Lay out your exercise clothes the night before, to help get you started and remove another barrier.

Where?

Many people find that it is difficult to find the time to exercise. If you can exercise at home, you may cut down on the time needed to exercise. Taking a walk early in the morning means only one shower and no travel time to the gym. Use your home exercise equipment or enjoy walking in your neighborhood, a local mall, park district facility, school track or gym.

When?

Studies have shown that people are more likely

to stick with their exercise plan if they exercise early in the morning. Daily life issues are less likely to intrude on your early morning routine. I personally like to exercise first thing, since I am not awake enough to notice. You may find that you can fit in exercise at lunch time at work. Put dinner in the oven and hit the treadmill to de-stress after your day. Or perhaps evenings after the kids go to bed is "your time." If you do strength training at home, you may find it easy to do while you are watching your favorite television show.

Exercise and anti-hypertensive medications

Some medications for hypertension will alter your response to exercise. Please check with your physician for any cautions about the type of exercise you can perform.

Exercise resources
Books
Strong Women Stay Young, Miriam Nelson, Bantam Books, 1997
Strong Women Stay Slim, Miriam Nelson, Bantom Books, 1999
Exercise: A Guide from the National Institute on Aging, National Institute on Aging.
Stretching, 20th Anniversary Edition, Bob and Jean

Anderson, Shelter Publications, 2000

Magazines
Shape
Self
Fitness
Prevention

Web sites
http://nihseniorhealth.gov/exercise/toc.html
Resources, free books, and an exercise video for
seniors.

http://www.cdc.gov/nccdphp/dnpa/physical/index.htm .
Physical fitness resources from the Centers on
Disease Control and Prevention.

http://www.collagevideo.com
Online catalogue of exercise videos.

http://dynamixmusic.com
CDs to energize your exercise routine.

For more current resources, see our web site at:
http://DASHdiet.org/exercise.htm

Chapter 6 DASH board

1. Plan to do some exercise each day.
2. Plan for a mix of aerobic, strength, flexibility, and balance exercises.
3. You may need to exercise 60 minutes per day if you are trying to lose weight.
4. Do exercise that you enjoy. You are more likely to keep it going.
5. Morning exercise may help avoid schedule conflicts.
6. Consider your personality type in choosing exercise programs.
7. Exercising at home may fit a hectic schedule.
8. Invest in your health. Buy equipment that allows you to exercise at home.
9. Stay hydrated while you exercise.
10. Even small bouts of exercise can have health benefits.

Tracking my Personal DASH Diet Action Plan:

What exercises will I incorporate into my routine, how long, and how often?

_____, _____ minutes, _____ x/week

_____, _____ minutes, _____ x/week

_____, _____ minutes, _____ x/week

Where will I do these exercise?

_____

_____

What time of day will I exercise?

_____

What equipment do I need?

_____

_____

Additional activities I enjoy:

_____

_____

What will keep me motivated?

_____

_____

Chapter 7 The DASH Diet and Other Health Concerns

People who have high blood pressure often have other health concerns. They may have type 2 diabetes or metabolic syndrome. Hypertension is associated with increased risk of other cardiovascular diseases such as atherosclerosis, congestive heart failure, stroke, and coronary artery disease. Fortunately the DASH diet can improve health for people with any of these conditions.

Diabetes

If you have type 1 diabetes (also known as insulin-dependent or juvenile) you should consult with your Registered Dietitian before making any changes in your diet. You need to be sure that you are coordinating your intake with your insulin and your activity schedule.

People who have type 2 diabetes (also known as non-insulin dependent or adult-onset) can usually follow the DASH diet and improve their blood sugar control. The high fiber intake can result in lower blood sugar. Many of the key minerals found in the DASH foods may be associated with improved sensitivity to insulin. This can reduce the need for medication or supplemental insulin and slow the progression of the disease. All of the key DASH foods are beneficial for people with diabetes. Whole grains, fruits, vegetables, low fat dairy, and even nuts are known to have special benefits for improving health for people with diabetes. Many dietitians have found that nuts improve glucose control in people with diabetes. The fiber in whole grains, fruits and vegetables can slow the absorption of sugar, avoiding large swings in blood glucose. Fruits and vegetables are rich in antioxidants which may be associated with reduction in complications from diabetes. Choosing low-fat or nonfat dairy, lean meats and poultry help reduce the risk of developing high cholesterol. Since people with diabetes are at higher risk for heart disease, the DASH diet is especially important. Weight loss and exercise have been shown to be able to reduce the risk of developing type 2 diabetes or reversing mild diabetes. The entire DASH action plan supports having good health even with diabetes.

Metabolic Syndrome

Dietary advice gets more complicated when high blood pressure gets mixed up with high triglycerides or elevated blood sugars. This gets into territory that may be diagnosed as Metabolic Syndrome or Syndrome X. (A syndrome, unlike a disease, involves a condition where not all of the symptoms are required for diagnosis.) A hallmark of Metabolic Syndrome is insulin resistance or the inability to properly utilize insulin. People with insulin resistance may have their symptoms worsened by a high refined carbohydrate diet. In order to get the best results from the DASH program, they may want to make some slight adjustments, while still remaining true to the DASH principles.

Insulin resistance is a condition where the body does not respond well to its own insulin. Blood sugars remain elevated longer than normal after a meal. To compensate, the body pumps out extra insulin in an attempt to reduce blood sugar. The extra insulin induces the body to produce more cholesterol, and plumps up fat cells (especially in our abdomen). Instead of storing sugar in our muscles for quick energy, we store the sugar in our fat cells where it is converted into fat. Our liver also tries to clean up extra blood sugar by converting it into triglycerides (more fat). Our body packages the triglycerides into vehicles that soak up cholesterol

> **Diagnosis of Metabolic Syndrome**
>
> 3 or more of the following:
> 1. Waist circumference higher than 40 inches for men or 35 inches for women.
> 2. Triglycerides higher than 150.
> 3. HDL < 40 for men, or <50 for women.
> 4. Blood pressure higher than 130/85 without medication.
> 5. Fasting glucose greater than 110.

from the HDL (good cholesterol). This shrinks the HDL, reducing its ability to clean up cholesterol in the arteries and increasing the risk of heart disease. Insulin resistance is considered to be a pre-diabetic condition.

Contrary to much of the healthy eating advice in the media, people who have Metabolic Syndrome are likely to have their health hurt by a high carbohydrate, low fat diet. The DASH diet is moderate in both carbohydrates and fats. With a few extra guidelines, it will allow someone with metabolic syndrome to enjoy all the benefits of DASH, improve the way their body metabolizes sugar, and perhaps stave off the onset of type 2 diabetes.

Insulin resistance may progress to a condition called "pre-diabetes," which is when the fasting blood sugar (glucose) measurement is between 110-125. People with metabolic syndrome will typically have blood sugars above 85. Although it still may be in the normal range," it is much higher than the optimal fasting blood sugar which is 70 - 85. Having a fasting blood sugar higher than 85 may indicate that you are not responding as well to insulin. Your triglycerides may also be elevated. When the body has had to produce extra insulin for several years, eventually it wears out its ability to produce enough insulin. Then the person will develop type 2 diabetes. Their body is producing insulin, but cannot produce enough to keep blood sugar under control.

DASH Diet Adjustments with Metabolic Syndrome or Type 2 Diabetes.

Avoiding high amounts of refined carbohydrates can support better glucose control in people with type 2 diabetes or with metabolic syndrome. For this reason, it may be easier to keep blood sugar under control if you limit refined carbohydrates. You can still include all of the key DASH foods such as fruits, vegetables, low fat dairy, nuts, beans, and lean meats. However, having piles of pasta, white rice, bagels and pretzels may not be so helpful.

What are refined carbohydrates? Any of the white grain foods are considered to be refined. They generally are very low in fiber, and low in minerals that are associated with improved blood pressure control. Refined grains include refined flour, white rice, and all the foods that are made from them. Bagels, pasta, pretzels, sweetened cereals, Italian bread, French bread, pastries, cakes and cookies all contain refined carbohydrates. Whole grains include whole wheat, brown rice, rye, oats, and pumpernickel. These grains are all brown, however, not all brown grain foods are made from 100% whole grains. Sometimes the brown color comes from caramel food coloring. It is important to check the food labels to be sure that all the flour in a bread or cereal comes from whole grains.

All starches, from refined and whole grains, are

broken down into glucose (the sugar in blood sugar measurements) during digestion. Therefore, both starch and sugar can elevate blood sugar. Even though starch is considered to be a complex carbohydrate, it does turn into glucose, and it happens relatively quickly with refined carbohydrates. So the question is not whether you should choose simple carbs or complex carbs, but rather, how can you include more high fiber carbs.

Foods that have more fiber tend to be broken down and absorbed more slowly than refined carbohydrates. This will result in less demand for the body to pump out extra insulin to keep blood sugar under control. This is certainly a nice benefit for people with type 2 diabetes or metabolic syndrome.

A lower (moderate) carbohydrate diet may also be necessary for weight reduction. If refined carbohydrates are limited, it will make it easier to include more servings of fruits, vegetables, and dairy foods. Key DASH nutrients such as calcium, potassium, magnesium, and fiber are not found in appreciable quantities in refined carbohydrates.

The DASH Diet Action Plan also includes recommendations for weight loss and exercise. Research has shown that these steps can help reverse or delay onset of prediabetes or clinical diabetes better than can medication.

Artery-blocking high cholesterol

The DASH diet has been shown to lower cholesterol. Cholesterol in the blood is found in several different forms. HDL (high density lipoprotein) is the good form of cholesterol. It is a form of "packaging" for cholesterol that actually cleans up the cholesterol in arteries. The LDL (low density lipoprotein) is the cholesterol package that tends to deposit cholesterol in the arteries. In general, we like to have more of the good cholesterol (HDL) and less of the bad cholesterol (LDL). Diet, weight reduction, and exercise as promoted in the DASH Diet Action Plan will support improving

Classifications of Blood Lipid Levels

Total Cholesterol
Desirable . . . . <200
Borderline high 200-239
High . . . . 240+
LDL cholesterol
Desirable with CVD . . . . <70
Optimal . . . . <100
Near or above optimal 100-129
Borderline high 130-159
High 160-189
Very high . . . . 190+
HDL cholesterol
Low . . . . <40
High (desirable) . . . . 60+
Triglycerides (triacylglyerols)
Normal . . . . <150
Borderline high 150-199
High 200-499
Very high . . . . 500+

cholesterol levels.

Specific nutrition recommendations for lowering cholesterol, include limited intake of dietary cholesterol, saturated and trans fats (discussed in chapter 9), increased intake of soluble fiber, soy foods, and plant stanols.

The high fiber in the DASH diet helps to lower cholesterol. Fiber that is especially good for helping to lower cholesterol is called functional fiber or soluble fiber. Some well-known examples include the beta-glucan in oats, pectin in apples, and psyllium found in Metamucil™. You can find a longer listing of these foods in Chapter 9.

Since the DASH diet encourages the use of low-fat or nonfat dairy foods, and lean meats, fish and poultry, there is little saturated fat which your body could use to make more cholesterol.

Another dietary change you could consider are plant stanols/sterols which are found in some margarines, including Benecol™ and Take Control™, and now are added to some juices. Research has shown that they can help lower cholesterol by up to 14%. Soy protein (and the fiber found in many soy products) can support lowering cholesterol as well.

Chapter 7 DASHboard

Metabolic Syndrome, Type 2 Diabetes

1. Avoid high carb, low fat diets. Choose moderate carb, moderate protein, moderate fat.
2. Add more fiber to your diet, from key DASH diet foods: whole grains, beans, nuts, vegetables and fruits.
3. Include 3 - 4 servings of low fat or nonfat dairy each day.
4. Add aerobic exercise to help burn off belly fat.
5. Add strength exercise to reduce insulin resistance.
6. Limit saturated fat and trans fat intake.

High Cholesterol

1. Limit intake of saturated fats, trans fats, and dietary cholesterol. Keep fat intake moderate.

Tracking my Personal DASH Diet Action Plan:

Current   **Target**
Fasting glucose _____   _____
Triglycerides   _____   _____

Changes I will make to improve my blood glucose
control: _____
_____

Changes I will make to lower my cholesterol and/or
triglycerides: _____
_____
_____

Chapter 8 Lifestyle Changes to Help Lower Blood Pressure

In this book we focus on healthy diet, weight loss, and exercise as lifestyle changes which help lower blood pressure. Additional key lifestyle changes that will help support lowering your blood pressure include smoking cessation and limiting alcohol consumption.

Alcohol

Healthy alcohol consumption is no more than one drink per day for women, and 2 drinks for men. In addition to raising blood pressure, alcohol is a source of empty calories, and can make it difficult to lose weight. Alcohol can cause elevated triglycerides, which is another heart disease risk. What counts as a drink?

- 12 ounces of beer
- 5 ounces of wine
- 1 ounces of 80-proof whiskey

Smoking

Smoking creates conditions which make it easier for cholesterol to stick onto the lining of the arteries. It facilitates blockage of arteries, which is no one's objective. In case you need a reminder, the National

Institutes of Health list the following reasons for quitting smoking:

- Reduce the risk of having a heart attack or stroke.
- Reduce the risk of getting lung cancer, emphysema, and other lung diseases.
- Climb stairs and walk without getting out of breath.
- Have younger skin, with fewer wrinkles.
- Eliminate morning cough.
- Reduce the number of coughs, colds, and earaches your child will have.
- Have more energy to pursue physical activities you enjoy.

When you quit smoking, you reduce by more than half your 1 year risk of heart disease. Quitting also reduces the risk of a second heart attack. Decide today that you no longer want to be a smoker.

Chapter 8 DASHboard

1. If you drink alcohol, do so in moderation. Limit to no more than one drink per day for women, two for men.
2. Stop smoking.

Tracking my Personal DASH Diet Action Plan:

I will limit myself to _____ drinks per day.

I will not start (or restart smoking) _____yes, _____no
I will quit smoking _____yes, _____ no
    by _____ (date)

Chapter 9 A Healthy Mix of Fats, Proteins and Carbs

Since the late 1980's the American public has been hearing the message that fat was bad. We were told to reduce the fat in our diet. They said that lowering fat would reduce our caloric intake and reduce our risk of heart disease and cancer. Companies rushed to produce fat-free products to meet the new consumer demand. Consumers feasted on SnackWell™ cookies, bagels and pretzels, which all were assumed to be healthier and to have less calories than the Oreos™, doughnuts, and Doritos™ which they replaced. We heard that Americans were eating too much meat, so we cut down or eliminated meat altogether. We were told that a high carb diet was the key to a healthier diet and would control weight. The percentage of fat calories in the American diet decreased, we consumed less protein and more carbs, while Americans became fatter.

Where did we get off track?

The truth about fat is much more complicated than just having less of it in our diet. And while we were eliminating fats, we eliminated too much protein, and overdid refined carbs. Getting on track with a healthy diet means reestablishing a balance of fats, protein, and carbs, and choosing healthy fats and carbs that are fiber-rich.

Choosing food that tastes great and is satisfying can help us eat less, while enjoying it more. Many low fat or low carb foods simply don't taste very good, and many have about the same calories as the foods they replace. Compared with high carb meals, moderate amounts of fat and protein help to provide satiety, improve flavor, and help us avoid overeating.

There are healthy fats that we want to include in our diets, and fats that we definitely need to limit. We want to make sure to get enough protein and fiber in our diets. The DASH diet supports this, and shows that these dietary changes help to lower blood pressure, reduce cholesterol, and provide a foundation for weight loss.

In this chapter you will learn which fats are healthy, good sources of these healthy fats, lean protein-rich foods, and how to choose carbs which are rich in more than just calories, and won't cause your blood sugar to soar.

Healthy Fats

All naturally occurring fats are mixtures. They contain fatty acids with different chain lengths, different amounts of saturation, and differing health effects. Some fats are essential, which means that we have to get enough of them in our diet. And some fats can make us healthier, while some can increase our risks for many diseases, especially heart disease.

Based on current knowledge, especially healthy fats include monounsaturated fats (olives, avocados, nuts) and omega-3 fatty acids (fish oils), while saturated fats are considered to be associated with increased risk for heart disease. Polyunsaturated fats fit in the middle, having some health promoting properties, and some potential risk.

Saturated versus unsaturated fats

One of the main classifications of fats has two categories, those that are saturated and those that are unsaturated. The unsaturated fats are further divided into monounsaturated and polyunsaturated fats. Saturation refers whether or not there is a full complement of hydrogen on the fat. Saturated fats (SFAs) have all the hydrogen they can possibly have; that is, they are "saturated" with hydrogen. Monounsaturated fats (MUFAs) are missing hydrogen in one spot, and polyunsaturated fats (PUFAs) are missing hydrogen in two or more spots. The PUFAs can be further divided as to where the unsaturation points occur, such as omega-3 and omega-6 fatty acids.

The MUFAs and PUFAs are liquids, while most saturated fats are solids. In order to turn liquid fats, such as corn oil or soybean oil into a solid fat to make margarine or shortening, it has to be hydrogenated. This makes the fat more saturated. The process of hydrogenating the oils can create trans fatty acids, which are considered to increase heart disease risk.

In general, most saturated fats, including trans fatty acids, are associated with increased risk of developing high blood cholesterol. Guidelines for healthy eating encourage people to get less saturated and hydrogenated fats in their diet. Monounsaturated fats are considered to be heart healthy and are encouraged in the diet. The omega-3 fatty acids are also especially heart healthy, and can be included in moderation. Polyunsaturated fats do not cause elevation in cholesterol levels and so are also relatively heart healthy.

The best recommendations are to keep fat at a moderate level (between 25 - 35 percent of total calories), by choosing lean meats, fish and poultry, low-fat and nonfat dairy products (to reduce saturated fat intake), include fish in your diet a few times a week (to increase omega-3 fatty acids), include moderate amounts of oils rich in monounsaturated fats, as well as nuts and seeds, limit foods containing hydrogenated fats, and limit or avoid fried foods.

More on fats and health

Both MUFAs and PUFAs help to lower cholesterol. MUFAs have an added benefit, since they do not lower the "good cholesterol," known as HDL. PUFAs can lower good cholesterol at the same time as they lower the bad cholesterol. They arc also a little less stable and may be susceptible to oxidation, which is undesirable. We need to get enough of these essential fats, but we don't want to overdo it.

A special type of PUFA is the omega-3 fatty

acids, such as those found in fish oils. The key fats are also known as DHA and EPA. Studies have shown that people who consume more fatty fish or fish oil supplements are less likely to die from heart disease, and possibly are less likely to develop cancer. Other potential benefits from fish oils include reducing the risk of developing diabetes, reducing the clotting tendencies of blood, reducing depression, and reducing inflammation in the body. Omega-3 fatty acids are also found in plant oils such as flaxseed and walnuts, but current research suggests that little of these fatty acids are converted into the healthy DHA and EPA.

I am not recommending for or against taking fish oil supplements. Any supplementation should be discussed with your physician and a registered dietitian. If you are taking blood thinners, like warfarin (Coumadin) or Plavix, fish oil could make you more likely to develop a bleeding problem or be susceptible to a hemorrhagic stroke. Many other over-the-counter medications or supplements, such as aspirin, vitamin E, garlic, and ginko biloba, inhibit blood clotting, so adding fish oil supplements could increase the risk of bleeding problems or stroke. Some studies have shown a negative interaction of fish oil supplements with certain diabetic medications. If you want to use fish oil supplements, be sure to discuss it with your physician (and a registered dietitian).

Food Sources of Fats
There are many reasons for including various

types of fat in our diets. When choosing which fats to add to foods or choosing foods which naturally contain fats, we can consider taste, cost, stability to heat, and health effects.

Saturated fats

Animal foods, including beef, pork, and dairy are the largest source of saturated fats in the typical American diet. However, today the beef and pork industries are producing leaner animals, and much leaner cuts of meat. Many reduced or nonfat dairy

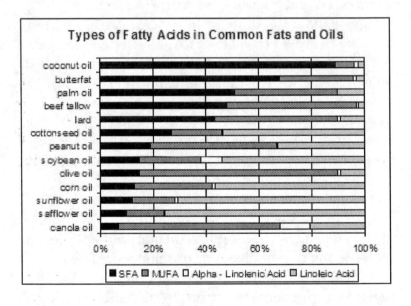

Types of Fatty Acids in Common Fats and Oils

foods allow us to add calcium to our diets without overdoing saturated fat.

And, as the above chart shows, saturated fats do not come just from animal foods. Coconut oil and palm oil are high in saturated fats. After coconut oil, butterfat has the highest percentage of saturated fat. You can make a big impact on your cholesterol by replacing full fat dairy foods with non-fat or reduced fat products, such as non-fat frozen yogurt, reduced fat cheese, non-fat cottage cheese, and skim milk.

It may be a surprise to many people that there are many types of beef and pork that are quite lean today and can be part of a heart healthy diet. To help you select lean cuts, a detailed comparison of fat content and calories of various meats, fish, and poultry are listed in Appendix A.

Monounsaturated fats

Olive oil and canola oil are the best known rich sources of monounsaturated fats. Olive oil contains slightly more MUFA

> **High fat, but not as high calorie as you think . . .**
>
> Olives, 5 small . . . . . 20 Cal
> Avocado, 1 ounce . . 50 Cal

than canola, but also contains slightly more SFA. Nuts and seeds and their oils are other good sources of MUFAs. If you like peanut butter, I recommend using the natural versions, which are not hydrogenated. Be sure to keep natural peanut butter in the refrigerator after opening, to avoid rancidity. And keep nut intake under control. A serving is just 1/4 cup of nuts. One serving has the protein of 1 ounce of meat, and the calories of 3 ounces.

Polyunsaturated fats

Soy and corn oil are the most popular sources of

polyunsaturated fats (PUFAs). Safflower, cottonseed, and sunflower are other readily available sources of PUFAs. There is a new variety of safflower which is high in oleic acid, which is a MUFA, so you may soon see safflower oil that is rich in MUFAs. The two essential fatty acids are PUFAs, linolenic and linoleic acids.

Omega-3 fatty acids

Flaxseed oil is the best known plant source of the omega-3 fatty acids. Soy and walnuts are also good plant sources. The plant oils provide alpha-linolenic acid (ALA), which is an essential fatty acid. The body converts some ALA into DHA and EPA, which are found in cold-water fatty fish, and are the key health-promoting omega-3 fats. It is believed that only small amounts of plant omega-3 fats get turned into DHA and EPA, so fish remains the best source. (Please see Appendix B for a list of common fish sources and their omega-3 content.) Flaxseed oil is very susceptible to rancidity, so if you decide to use it, be sure that it is stored in a cold, dark place, and buy small quantities, so that you don't store it for long periods.

Hydrogenated fats

Shortening and margarine are two common sources of hydrogenated fats. In general, any vegetable oil that has been turned into a solid, is hydrogenated. Food labels are a good source of information on hydrogenated fats in food. Look for the terms hydrogenated fats or partially-hydrogenated fats in the ingredient list. Most baked goods, such as snack crackers, pastries, and cookies are rich in these types of fats. Labeling for trans fatty acids is being phased in on the Nutrition Facts panel of the food label.

Protein

Protein is a basic building block for our body. It forms the basis of our muscles, skin, and organs. Specialized proteins act as hormones, while others act as enzymes to help to digest and metabolize our

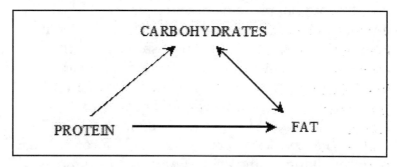

food. Proteins help to carry nutrients such as fats and minerals in our blood. As seen in the previous chart, we can convert carbs and protein into fat, or fat and protein into carbs; however, we cannot make protein from fat or carbohydrates. We have to get enough protein in our diet to maintain or build muscle and keep our metabolism high.

Protein Quality

Amino acids are the building blocks of all

proteins in our bodies. Some amino acids are essential, meaning that we have to obtain them from food, and some amino acids can be made in the body by transforming one of the essential amino acids into a nonessential one. In general, animal proteins are better quality than vegetable protein. The quality is based on whether the protein has all of the essential amino acids in the right proportion. Fortunately for vegetarians, having vegetable protein from a variety of sources improves the total protein quality of the diet. Many vegetable proteins are complementary to each other by filling in the gaps for inadequate amino acids from other foods.

Most animal proteins provide all of the essential amino acids in the right amounts. The proteins in eggs, dairy, meat, poultry, and fish are all high quality proteins. Isolated soy protein is considered to be a high quality plant protein. Other plants proteins such as corn, wheat, and beans are incomplete proteins, but still are beneficial in a diet that is balanced with "complementary" proteins that supply lacking amino acids. Some good examples of complementary plant proteins include rice and beans, corn and beans, wheat and corn, and peanut butter and wheat bread. It is interesting that many of these foods are often paired in ethnic cuisines. We often find rice and beans in dishes in Caribbean and Latin American cuisines. Chinese, Japanese, and Indian dishes often combine beans and rice.

How much protein do we need?
Many popular diet books have promoted high

consumption of protein foods. This conflicts with much of the advice that we have received over the past several decades, urging Americans to reduce the amount of protein in their diets. The DASH diet is a moderate plan that emphasizes adequate protein. Studies show that getting enough protein helps to lower blood pressure.

So then, how much do we need? The new DRIs (Dietary Recommended Intake) for protein says that it should be 15 to 35% of your calories, or minimally 0.4 g protein per pound of weight (or more accurately, 0.8 g per kilogram). The amount of protein that you need is proportional to your weight, so if you are on a weight loss plan, you will want to maintain (or possibly increase) your protein intake, while cutting out empty carbs. A weight maintenance versions of the DASH diet will probably provide about 20% of calories from protein. People who are on a DASH weight loss plan will have a higher percentage of total calories from protein.

What does this mean in real-life terms? If you weigh 154 pounds, the minimum amount of protein that you would need is 56 grams. You can get 58 grams of protein by consuming 2 glasses of milk and six ounces of meat, fish, or poultry. If you add six servings of grains and 4 servings of vegetables, you will add another 26 grams of protein. So, you can see that it isn't very difficult to get the amount of protein that you need in a day.

Food sources of protein

Where do we find protein in our diet? Most of the food groups, except for fruits and fats, contain protein. Grains, vegetables, dairy foods, meats, fish, and poultry, along with eggs, legumes, nuts and seeds all contain protein. The richest sources are meats, fish, poultry, and eggs. And, in general, animal sources of protein have the best quality, with grains having poor quality protein. The following list shows the amount of protein in different types of foods.

Protein Content of Foods		
Food Group	Serving Size	Protein Grams
Grains	1 slice bread, 1/2 cup cooked grains such as pasta, or oatmeal, 1/2 English muffin or bun, 1/4 bagel, ⅓ cup rice	3
Vegetables	1/2 cup cooked vegetables, 1 cup raw leafy greens	2
Nuts	1 oz or 1/4 cup	7
Beans	1/2 cup	7
Dairy	1 cup milk, 8 oz yogurt, 1 oz cheese	8
Meat	1 oz meat, poultry or fish, 1 egg, 1/4 cup nuts	7

Low fat and lean protein-rich foods

The best protein sources are low in saturated fats and rich in vitamins and minerals. This includes lean meats, fish, poultry, low-fat and nonfat dairy foods, soy products, beans, nuts, and egg whites.

When the relationship of heart disease with cholesterol and high-fat animal foods was first noted, the prevailing wisdom told us to reduce our intake of red meat and many dairy foods. People eliminated or reduced red meat consumption. But now, many of my clients tell me that they are tired of having "the same old chicken" for dinner every night. The great news is that there are many alternatives. There are a variety of lean meats, and low fat or nonfat dairy foods available. Healthy diets can include red meat and dairy foods that are low in fat, along with poultry, fish and vegetable protein sources.

The key to leaner meats is to look for cuts that are called loin or round. Sirloin, tenderloin, and loin chops (including NY strip steaks) are all lean cuts. Another helpful tip is to choose select cuts. Prime and choice cuts have more fat and calories. Fortunately, select is the grade of meat that is available in most grocery stores. When you are in better restaurants you are more likely to find choice or prime cuts. You may decide to choose seafood if you want a lower fat restaurant choice. Prime rib would be a very fatty beef choice. Beef tenderloin is a lower fat option and equally tender and flavorful.

Within each type of protein food group, there are likely to be many lean choices to keep you from getting bored with your meals. If you want to have beef, top loin chops and tenderloin make good steak-type choices. You can make a burger with 95% lean ground sirloin, that is almost as lean as the same amount of white chicken meat. Pork is generally lean. Even ham is now a great low fat choice. If you like the taste of barbecued ribs, try pork chops with barbecue sauce, for a meatier, lighter choice. Skinless chicken or turkey breast make tasty low fat choices. Surprisingly, most of the ground turkey in grocery stores contains added turkey fat and ground skin, and often has more fat than lean ground beef. Most fish and seafood is low fat, with some being extremely low fat. Expand your repertoire, and break out of your dinner-time rut, with protein choices that won't contribute to a cholesterol problem.

Appendix A lists many types of meat, poultry and fish that will give you more lean choices at home or in restaurants. The tables provide calories, fat grams and more.

Reduced fat dairy products also are terrific protein sources. While many low-fat baked goods have calories as high as the original high-fat foods, reduced fat dairy foods give you a big payoff in reducing the calorie and saturated fat content of your diet. For example, skim milk (now called fat free milk) only has 90 calories compared with 150 for whole milk (with 3.5% butterfat). It has just as much protein and calcium, without the fat.

Plant protein foods are often fat-free. Beans and grains have little or no fat. Nuts and seeds are high fat protein foods. So it is helpful to watch your serving sizes when eating nuts. Nuts are rich in minerals, fiber, and monounsaturated fats, so there are substantial health benefits from including moderate amounts of nuts in your diet.

Fat content is not the only factor you should use in making protein choices. Fatty cold-water fish is a good sources of omega-3 fatty acids. Even though shrimp is high in cholesterol, it is very low in saturated fat and in calories and is considered to be heart healthy. Beef is very rich in minerals and vitamins. A 3-ounce serving of lean beef contains only 10% of the daily value (DV) for calories, but 50% of the protein, 39% of the zinc, 37% of the vitamin B_{12}, 16% of vitamin B_6, and 14% of the iron. Milk, yogurt, and cheese are all rich in calcium. Beans are rich in soluble fiber and contribute iron and zinc. Nuts and seeds contribute fiber and minerals. Fat content is an important consideration, but don't make that your only cue. You have more good protein choices than you think.

The DASH plan encourages you to include a variety of low-fat protein foods in your diet. Each day we should include about 6 ounces from the meat group (or plant protein) and 2 - 3 servings of low fat dairy foods. And we should include 4 - 5 servings of nuts or beans each week.

Carbohydrates

What is all the talk about "bad" carbs and "good" carbs? In general, good carbs do not cause your blood sugar to shoot up, and they usually are rich sources of vitamins, minerals, and fiber. Bad carbs may provide empty calories, without bringing much nutritional value.

The concept of identifying how likely carbohydrate-rich foods are to cause blood sugar (glucose) to rise is called glycemic index (GI). It is considered by many experts to be an important consideration for weight loss and for managing blood sugar. Simple sugars and starch are easy for the body to break down and absorb. And most starch gets digested to glucose, which is directly related to rises in glucose in the blood.

Foods which can cause blood sugar to rise are identified as high glycemic index foods. Low GI foods tend to have high fiber content. People with high blood pressure are likely to be sensitive to high GI foods.

The DASH diet is rich in carbs loaded with fiber, having a low glycemic index. When you eat 4 - 5 servings of fruits and 4 - 5 servings of vegetables, you automatically add lots of fiber to your diet. Whole grains are another great way to add fiber. And the DASH diet recommends 4 - 5 servings per week of nuts and beans, adding yet more fiber. The typical DASH diet at 2000 Calories contains over 31 grams of fiber.

Fiber

Fiber has additional benefits beyond helping to keep blood sugar on a more even keel after meals. Actually there are two types of fiber, one that promotes regularity, and another type that has some special health benefits. The fiber known as "roughage" which helps to keep us regular, is called "insoluble fiber." The other type is called "soluble fiber" or the newer term, "functional fiber."

Roughage helps to speed the flow of wastes through our digestive tract, and can help keep us

Good Sources of Fiber		
	soluble fiber	total fiber
Apple, unpeeled	.4	3.0
Pear, unpeeled	.7	4.6
Raspberries, 1/2 cup	.3	2.6
Prunes, 5	1.1	3.1
Avocado, 1/2	1.2	3.8
Sweet potato, 1/2 cup	.5	1.9
Broccoli, 2 stalks	.2	1.8
Carrots, 1/2 cup	.4	1.9
Spaghetti sauce, 1/2 cup	.6	3.0
Kidney beans, 1/2 cup	1.0	4.5
All bran cereal, ⅓ cup	.7	8.1
Oatmeal, 3/4 cup	1.2	2.7

"regular." It may also help reduce the risk of colon

cancer. It is found in the skins and pulp of fruits, the seeds in berries, the outer covering of whole grains, and in vegetables.

Soluble fiber has many interesting properties. It also helps to promote regularity by making the waste more bulky, softer, and easier to move through the intestines. It also thickens the digested food in our small intestines, so that absorption of sugars is slowed. It can soak up cholesterol so that it gets eliminated rather than being absorbed. Soluble fiber is found in oats and barley, fruits (especially apples, pears, and oranges), beans and lentils, and in vegetables.

Even though most Americans get more food than they need each day, most of us get way too little fiber. Guidelines suggest that we should get at least 25 grams of fiber each day. Most of the people that I see in my private practice get less than 12 grams of fiber per day. Beyond salads and potatoes, most of us are missing out on a variety of vegetables with our on-the-go eating. Many people say they forget to eat fresh fruit, so they stop buying it. Bagels have replaced whole grain cereals for a quick, on-the-run breakfast. And beans and lentils are not even on the radar screen. With the DASH diet, getting sufficient fiber in your diet is all part of the plan. You don't even have to think about it.

Introducing More Fiber Into Your Diet
Many of us have gotten used to consuming a low fiber diet. In order to help your body adjust to

higher amounts of fiber (with all those DASH fruits and vegetables), it can be helpful to go slowly. As we age, some people find that high fiber foods cause discomfort, and they experience intestinal bloating or gas. The gradual approach may allow your body to better adjust to fiber. Try to add 1 - 2 extra fruits or vegetables to your daily intake, and then hold at that level for several days. Then increase again. If you find that you are still uncomfortable, you may want to try one of the fiber digesting supplements. There are several brands on the market, including Beano.

It is very important to increase your intake of fluid when you add more fiber. You must get at least 8 glasses of fluid per day. A high fiber diet without plenty of fluid will still leave you constipated. (If you have congestive heart failure, consult with your physician and a registered dietitian before making any changes in your diet, both in terms of the amount of fluid and in the amount of fiber.)

Chapter 9 DASHboard

1. A balanced approach to fat, protein, and carbs is important for health and for a healthy weight.
2. Choose unsaturated fats, especially MUFAs and omega-3 PUFAs. Limit SFA.
3. Good sources of MUFAs are olive oil, canola oil, nuts and avocados.
4. Good sources of omega-3 fatty acids are fish, such as tuna, salmon, sardines, and herring.
5. High fat animal foods are the primary source of saturated fats, which should be limited.
6. For lean meats, choose "select" meats with the words "loin" or "round" in their name.
7. Low fat and nonfat dairy are low in calories and saturated fats.
8. High fiber foods may help to control hunger, help to lower cholesterol, and reduce the risk for certain types of cancer.

Tracking my Personal DASH Diet Action Plan:
Food sources of healthy fats I will choose, include:

_____

_____

_____

Lean or low fat protein foods I will choose include:

_____

_____

_____

High fiber foods I will choose, include:

_____

_____

_____

Chapter 10 Beyond a DASH of Salt – Minerals That Help to Lower Blood Pressure

Doctors have known for many years that moderation of salt intake can help many people lower blood pressure. It has been less well known that several other minerals can help reduce blood pressure when we include more of them in our diets. Diets that are rich in calcium, potassium, and magnesium, in particular, have been shown to lower blood pressure, and the majority of Americans do not get enough. Fortunately, this plan will assure that you meet your needs, since foods rich in these minerals are the foundation of the DASH diet.

A DASH of Salt

Everyone has heard that lowering salt will lower blood pressure. Recently there has been some controversy about this broad statement. Some people may be more sensitive than others to the effects of salt or sodium. (We talk about salt almost interchangeably with sodium, since it is the major contributor of sodium to our diets.) And there are several other minerals, such as potassium, calcium, and magnesium, which play into the equation.

The original DASH investigation used a moderate level of sodium, 3,200 mg per day, well above the current recommendations. With the DASH diet, blood pressure was lowered significantly, even at this moderately high intake of sodium. But the question remained, what if the salt level were lower, would there be further improvements in blood pressure control? Recent DASH studies have shown that, in fact, the lower the salt intake with the DASH diet, the more the blood pressure declined. So, yes, watching your sodium intake is still a good thing.

Many studies have shown that people around the world who consume more sodium have higher blood pressures. This sensitivity increases with age. Societies where people do not consume any salt have almost no hypertension, and blood pressure does not increase with age. (In general these people also have low weight, low alcohol consumption, and high levels of physical activity.)

Typically, African Americans are quite sensitive to salt, and blacks have higher rates of hypertension than whites and Hispanics in the U. S. In the DASH study that looked at lower salt levels, blacks, and especially black women, responded better than whites to salt restriction.

Interestingly, as much as it seems like gospel that we should all try to lower our sodium intake, there are some studies in the U. S. which have shown that low intake of sodium is associated with shorter lifespan. Further, some people may actually be at risk of developing increased blood pressure if they adopt a diet that is overly restrictive in sodium. This includes people who have a cluster of symptoms known as metabolic syndrome, which include overweight, high blood pressure, high triglycerides, low HDL (good) cholesterol and high LDL (bad) cholesterol, and carrying excess weight around the waist or upper body.

Beyond Salt – Calcium, Potassium, and Magnesium

Sodium isn't the only mineral that helps with controlling blood pressure. Calcium, magnesium and potassium are all involved in helping to regulate blood pressure. And their relationship with blood pressure is generally positive. That is, getting more of these minerals in your diet helps to lower blood pressure.

Calcium

Calcium has many interesting health benefits beyond strengthening bones. People who consume more calcium in their diets have lower blood pressure, weigh less, have less body fat, and have lower risk of developing type 2 diabetes. The DASH diet encourages at least 2 - 3 servings a day of low-fat or nonfat dairy foods. More servings are needed to get the recommended amount of calcium for people over 50. It is preferable to include 3 - 4 daily servings of dairy to get 1200 mg of calcium per day, which is the RDA for people over 50.

The news about all the extra health benefits of

dairy is really very exciting. How nice to be able to add foods into your diet that have such positive benefits. Over the last 30 years, Americans' consumption of milk has declined dramatically. Many researchers have noted a connection between decreased consumption of milk and increased rates of obesity and hypertension. It is important to choose low-fat or nonfat dairy foods, as consumption increases. The fat in milk is butterfat, and it is one of the highest saturated fat foods. Skim (nonfat) milk, reduced fat or nonfat cheese, and nonfat yogurt are all great additions to your diet. If you find skim milk too "watery" you may find that low carb nonfat milk is much richer tasting, and has a "whiter" color than regular skim milk.

If you are lactose intolerant, you can find lactose-free milk. The lactose in yogurt has already been broken down by the bacteria that turn milk into yogurt, making it a great choice. Most cheese is also very low in lactose, having less than 1 gram per serving. If you must avoid milk, make sure to choose yogurts with vitamin D added, or consider taking a multivitamin. Vitamin D is essential for absorbing calcium, but it is not found in cheese and most yogurts.

There are many vegetables that are good sources of calcium, and many plant-based foods, such as soy milk, that are formulated to be good sources of calcium, so that even a vegan diet can provide plenty of calcium.

Potassium

A large world-wide study (Intersalt) showed that if potassium was high in relation to sodium, blood pressure was lower. Unfortunately, most Americans do not get enough potassium in their diets. One of the benefits of the DASH diet is that it will automatically increase intake of potassium while minimizing added salt. The DASH diet encourages 4 - 5 servings of fruits and 4 - 5 servings of vegetables each day, many of which are rich sources of potassium.

Potassium allows the body to get rid of extra fluid so that the heart doesn't have to pump too hard, thereby allowing blood pressure to stay low. It is also important for regulating the heart beat. Good sources of potassium include most fruits and vegetables, especially oranges, bananas, potatoes, and tomatoes, as shown in the table at the end of this chapter. High amounts of dietary potassium can counteract some of the effects of higher sodium.

Some people are on blood pressure medication that can interfere with excreting potassium, and their doctors may recommend limiting potassium intake. Even though there are many health benefits of potassium, do not use the advice given here to override your doctor's recommendation. If you would like to adopt the DASH diet and have been cautioned about too much potassium, be sure to discuss this with your physician.

Magnesium

Magnesium is another important mineral for keeping blood pressure under control. And, most Americans do not get enough magnesium in their diets. Whole grains are great sources of magnesium, as are nuts, and some vegetables and fruits. The tables at the end of this chapter will show you which foods are rich in magnesium.

Shaking the Salt Habit

Many people feel that it is difficult to limit sodium, since it is an important source of flavor in our diet. Salt has been very important throughout human history and many ancient villages were situated to be close to salt deposits. In addition to flavoring foods, salt was important in preserving foods in northern climates. The ancient Romans paid their soldiers in salt; the Latin word for salt is the root of the English word, salary.

We don't have to give up all salt, but we can make significant reductions though some easy substitutions.

1. Choose frozen vegetables instead of canned. No salt is added to frozen vegetables.
2. Choose low- or no-salt canned vegetables. Currently there is no frozen alternative to canned tomato products. Most have relatively high added salt. You can find low-salt or no-added-salt versions of most tomato products.
3. Avoid salt products earlier in the day if you are going to have tomato products with salt in them

at dinner. For example, if you are having spaghetti with canned tomato sauce at dinner, avoid canned tuna or other salted foods at breakfast and lunch.

4. Limit cured meats, such as bacon, ham, sausage, hot dogs, etc. The salt that is added to these foods is necessary to preserve the meat. So limit these foods to once a week or less.

5. Limit canned soups. Make your own soups without added salt.

6. Choose lower salt cheeses such as Swiss or Lorraine. Use smaller amounts of high salt cheeses. Read labels to check the sodium content of various cheeses.

7. Using fresh fruit as a dessert instead of baked goods such as cookies, naturally reduces sodium while increasing fruit servings.

8. Try cucumbers covered in a sweet vinegar such as rice wine vinegar, red wine vinegar, or balsamic vinegar rather than pickles.

9. Limit olives and capers.

10. Indulge your salt craving with a 1/2 ounce servings of potato chips instead of a "Grab Bag™" sized serving. You will limit your sodium to only 90 milligrams, and limit the weight consequences, since this portion only has 75 calories. (Yes, this is a surprise. You can include some salted snacks without overdoing sodium.)

11. Choose seasoning mixes without salt, such as lemon pepper mix, or other seasoning flavors.

12. Forget about salting your fries. If you need

seasoning, try spice mixes. At restaurants where you don't have options, you may find that you don't even miss the salt. (And limiting fries is a good thing for reducing calories and added fats.)

13. Reduce salt in canned beans by rinsing well in water. If you have the time, let them soak in water for 30 minutes to eliminate more sodium.

14. Choose lentils for your bean dish if you would normally use canned beans. Lentils don't require the long overnight soaking like dry beans.

DASH Diet Mineral-rich Foods

Since we don't eat minerals, we need to meet our dietary requirements from foods. The following lists show you which foods are rich in the key blood pressure-lowering minerals. You will also see that these foods are the key DASH foods.

Potassium-rich foods

Vegetables
asparagus
artichoke
bamboo shoots
beets
broccoli
Brussels
sprouts
carrots
beans
cauliflower
celery
kale
mushrooms
okra
potatoes
pumpkin
seaweed
spinach
turnip greens
squash
(winter)
sweet potato
tomatoes

Fruits
apricots
avocado
banana
cantaloupe
grapefruit
honeydew
kiwifruit
orange
prunes
strawberries
tangerine
dried fruits
apple
apricots
dates
pear
peach

Cereals and Breads
bran cereals
Mueslix
pumpernickel
bread

Nuts
almonds
brazil nuts
cashews
chestnuts
filberts
hazelnuts
peanuts
pecans
pumpkin seeds
sunflower
seeds
walnuts

Miscellaneous
coffee
molasses
tea
tofu

Magnesium-rich foods

Fruits and Vegetables	Whole Grains	Nuts
avocado	amaranth	pumpkin seeds
banana	barley	sunflower seeds
beet greens	buckwheat	sesame seeds
blackeye peas	bulgur	almonds
casava	granola	cashews
beans and lentils	millet	flax seeds
figs	oats	hazel nuts
okra	brown rice	brazil nuts
potatoes with skin	wild rice	peanuts
raisins	rye	walnuts
seaweed	triticale	pistacios
spinach	whole wheat bran	soybeans
Swiss chard		macadamia nuts
wax beans		pecans

Calcium rich foods

Dairy	Vegetables	Beans
milk	broccoli	soybeans
yogurt	kale	tofu
cottage cheese	bok choi	
cheese		

Chapter 10 DASHboard

1. Avoid salt. Limit canned and processed foods. Limit olives, pickles, and capers. Choose low salt cheeses. Limit cured meats, such as bacon, ham, and sausages.
2. Include lots of foods rich in potassium, calcium, and magnesium. These include fruits, vegetables, whole grains, dairy, and nuts.

Tracking my Personal DASH Diet Action Plan:

I will include the following foods in my diet:
Potassium-rich: _____

_____

Magnesium-rich: _____

_____

Calcium-rich: _____

_____

I will limit sodium by avoiding the following:

_____

_____

My low salt alternatives will be: _____

_____

_____

Chapter 11 Deciphering the Food Labels

Nutrition labels were developed to help people make nutritious food choices that would benefit their health. Many of the nutrients that are required to be displayed on the label can help people reduce their risk of developing or help manage some very common diseases and conditions, such as heart disease, hypertension, diabetes, and obesity. The key nutrients include calories, total fat, cholesterol, sodium, total carbohydrate, and protein.

For someone following the DASH diet, the Nutrition Facts panel can help with making good food choices. Choosing lean meat and poultry and low-fat dairy foods is easy when you can easily see how much fat is in the food, and which types are low in saturated fats. You can make low sodium choices, and look for high fiber foods – all based on the Nutrition Facts.

Specific information must be in the Nutrition Facts, panel, label, as shown here. In the follwoing sections we will go through the panel, step-by-step to explain all the components.

Serving size

First, you want to know how much is in a serving of the food. In this example, which is plain yogurt, the serving size is 1 cup, which is the amount in the entire container. If there are multiple servings in a container, the Nutrition Facts panel will key you in to this. For example, a bag of microwave popcorn might contain 2 or 3 servings. You need to check to be sure what serving size the calories and nutrients are based on.

Plain Yogurt

Nutrition Facts

Serving Size 1 cup (248 g)
Servings per container 1

Amount Per Serving	
Calories 150 Calories from Fat 35	

	% Daily Value*
Total Fat 4 g	6%
Saturated Fat 2.5 g	12%
Cholesterol 20 mg	7%
Sodium 170 mg	7%
Total Carbohydrate 17 g	6%
Dietary Fiber 0 g	
Sugars 17 g	
Protein 13g	

Vitamin A 4%	•	Vitamin C 6%
Calcium 40%	•	Iron 0%

*Percent Daily Values are based on a 2,000 calorie diet.

In general, for multi-serving packages, there are standardized serving sizes. However, it gets a little confusing when you have single-serving containers with different sizes. For example, the standard serving of potato chips is 1 ounce. However, if you have a 1/2 ounce bag of chips, that is a serving for that package. If you have a 11/2 ounce bag, that also is a serving for that package.

Cereals are one of the most challenging foods to judge a serving size. The standard serving size is 1 ounce. If you have a cereal that is full of air, it takes more in terms of volume to equal 1 (weight) ounce. With a very dense cereal, like Grape Nuts™, technically, a serving is only 1/4 cup, whereas the label shows 1/2 cup which is 2 ounces. If you have a

148

cup of Grape Nuts™, you are actually having 4 servings of cereal. It is very important to check the serving size.

Total calories and calories from fat

The total calories are related to the serving size. The calories from fat give you an idea of the nutrient density. Foods that are high in fat, but don't have a lot of vitamins, minerals, or protein, may be considered to have a low nutrient density. They bring lots of calories, but not much nutritional value. If someone eats a high fat diet, it is possible that he or she could be getting adequate calories, but still be malnourished. If you consume a lot of high fat foods, you may not be able to eat much and still stay within your target calorie range. So, go easy on the foods that have more than 30% of their calories from fat.

Nutrient composition

The next section gives you the grams of various nutrients in a serving, and the percent daily values. The daily values percentage can often be very confusing. Many people look at the percentage, and think that it represents the percent of that nutrient in the food. Using the yogurt example, the 4 grams of fat represent 6% of the requirement for a day, for a 2000 calories diet. It doesn't mean that 6% of the calories in the yogurt come from fat. In fact, since 35 of the 150 calories come from fat (from the top section), this means that 23% of the calories are from fat. A new requirement will add trans fat to the listing, if it is present in the food.

Sodium and occasionally potassium are found in this section. You, obviously, want to limit sodium and choose foods that are rich in potassium.

In the carbohydrate section you will find total carbohydrates, fiber and sugars. The part that isn't shown is mostly starch, which you can compute by subtracting fiber and sugar from the total carbohydrate value. Fibers may also be broken down further to show soluble fiber.

Additional vitamins and minerals with special public health concerns are shown in the bottom section of the Nutrition Facts panel. Vitamin C, Vitamin A, calcium, and iron content must be included on the label. Manufacturers may add additional vitamins and mineral content at this point.

Ingredients

Another requirement for food labels is that they must include the ingredient list. If you are concerned about cholesterol, you may want to go easy on foods that contain hydrogenated or partially hydrogenated fats.

The ingredient list is another way to check how much sugar has been added to a food. Some of the many terms which indicate sugar, include high fructose corn syrup, corn syrup, honey, molasses, dextrose, fructose, lactose, and more. Since ingredients must be listed in order by weight (from the highest to the lowest), having many sources of sugar can help the manufacturer disguise the importance of sugar in the overall product formula. The Nutrition Facts panel will provide better information on the amount of sugar in a specific food. Many healthy DASH diet foods naturally contain sugars (such as fruits, yogurt, and milk) and should not be avoided.

Chapter 11 DASHboard

1. Food labels help you limit intake of sodium, saturated and trans fats.
2. Read food labels closely to check serving size.
3. Use food labels to limit calories.
4. Use food labels to find foods rich in potassium and calcium.

Tracking my Personal DASH Diet Action Plan:

I will read food labels to choose healthy DASH diet foods:

Never ☐
Rarely ☐
Often ☐
I already read food labels ☐

Chapter 12 Vegetables for Picky Eaters

The following chapter reveals the "true confessions" of a picky eater and former vegetable-hater. As a child, the only cooked vegetables I would eat were sweet corn (really a grain and not a vegetable) and potatoes. Sometimes I would eat green beans or wax beans, but not often. I did like many raw vegetables, such as tomatoes, lettuce, carrots, and celery. But I would reject any of these foods if they were cooked. Now I am a fairly adventurous eater. What changed? First I got older. Children taste foods more intensely than adults. So, as we become older, we may find that foods which we didn't like as children, aren't quite so bad. And we may find that we actually *like* some of these previously "distasteful" foods. Check out your adult taste buds on new vegetables.

Another factor in our changing preferences is that we have changed how we cook vegetables. It is trendy to cook vegetables "tender-crisp" rather than boiling them until they are quite soft. This keeps the flavor milder and sweeter. Gentle microwaving and steaming are less likely to form the strong flavors that we associate with some members of the cabbage family such as broccoli and cauliflower, and also avoid mushy textures.

Many things contribute to an appreciation of vegetables. The following ideas have worked for me and for my patients. There will probably still be vegetables that you really can't "stomach," so don't feel like a failure if you are resistant to some. Our goal is just to expand your comfort zone. Several of the following suggestions are sure to click with you as you expand your palate.

Grow your meal.

A fun way to get more vegetables into your life is to plant some vegetables in your garden. Fresh foods taste better, and it is very satisfying to create something of value by growing your own food. There are many types of vegetables you can grow, even if you only have a small space. Try one or two, or try several for a real harvest bounty.

Peppers come in many colors and add adventure to your garden. Bell peppers in red, yellow, orange, ivory, and purple add as much color as flowering plants. The hotter peppers like red jalapeños and orange habañeros are a great way to spice up your plantings. Peppers are excellent sources of nutrients and antioxidants, such as carotenoids (orange, yellow and red colors) and vitamin C. The cool crunch adds extra texture to your salads and makes a colorful addition to an appetizer tray. Jalapeños add zest to fresh salsa made with tomatoes or fruit. You may get added health benefits from the capsaicin which puts heat into hot peppers.

Red cabbage looks like a big lush flower in your garden. It makes a great accent between your plants, and on the table. It adds color in salads, or braised for a succulent side dish. Broccoli is a fast grower, and can quickly produce a tender, mild vegetable for your dinner plate. Both red cabbage and broccoli are members of the cruciferous vegetable family, and are rich sources of vitamin C, beta carotene, and other substances that may help protect against cancer. When you pick them straight from the garden and eat them right away, there is less chance for losing storage-sensitive nutrients such as vitamin C.

Tomatoes are a perennial garden favorite, and produce fruit with much more flavor than store-bought tomatoes. New varieties, such as grape tomatoes, produce lavish harvests and are incredibly sweet. They add color and great flavor to your salads or simmered in sauces for your entrées. Tomatoes are rich in carotenoids, especially lycopene, which is a powerful antioxidant. Yellow tomatoes don't contain lycopene, but make colorful additions to your dinners and brighten up your garden. Tomatoes are great source of vitamin C.

You can sneak onions in between your flowers and vegetables, where they may protect your plants from insects. And, they can also protect you. The allium found in foods in the onion family may reduce the risk of several types of cancer. Other easy-to-grow choices from the onion family include chives, leeks, shallots and garlic. They add flavor to many types of foods to increase your dining pleasure, and they are good for you. Garlic has been shown to help reduce cholesterol, while it adds nuances to your sauces and salads.

Climbing vegetables can grow up a fence or a wall or a balcony rail. Green beans, wax beans, peas, and cucumbers add greenery to your yard, without taking up space. (And they stay cleaner when they are off the ground.) Fresh baby green beans or the skinny French *haricots verts* have a tenderness and sweetness you miss in the varieties from the store. Low in calories and good sources of vitamin C, beans are terrific additions to your summertime dinners. A wall of lettuce can be fun if you are handy. The lettuces grow in a bag filled with soilless growing medium, and peek out from the branches of a lattice. You won't need trips to the grocery store for fresh greenery. Darker colored lettuce can be a good source of carotenoids, vitamins E and K, as well as potassium.

If you have lots of space, you can add yellow crookneck squash and zucchini. Low calorie members of the squash family, they are terrific sliced in a salad or sautéed as a side dish. They can also be cut in chunks to be skewered for a shish kabob. The starchier winter squashes, will last further into the fall, and with their yellow color, they are obviously very rich in carotenoids, especially beta carotene. Roasted at a high temperature in the oven, their sweetness will complement a winter dinner.

Beans, beans, beans.

Most Americans are reluctant to add beans to their diet. (Here we are referring to legumes such as soy beans, kidney beans, lentils, and navy beans. Green beans don't count in this category.) Legumes are rich in vegetable protein and soluble fiber which lowers cholesterol. Some people don't know what to do with beans, some people don't like the flavor, and some people have texture aversions to beans. There are tricks to get around any of these concerns. If you don't like the texture or flavor of soy or other beans, there are some great soy-based meat substitutes available at your supermarket to make it easy for you to add the health benefits of beans to your diet. You may already be familiar with soy-based vegetarian burgers. Did you know that there are many other soy-based products, such as "chicken" nuggets, Buffalo wings, hot dogs, and even ground "meat?" These fit the bill for fast, easy meals that include all the advantages of soy, such as lowering cholesterol, improving the absorption of calcium, adding beneficial fiber, and providing phytochemicals which may help to lower your risk of some kinds of cancer. Women especially are looking for ways to incorporate soy into their diets, since it may help relieve some symptoms of menopause. Chocolate-based soy "milk" drinks provide another tasty way to add the benefits of soy to your day.

I will admit to not liking the unenhanced taste of soy. I spent several years working as a food scientist at a soy company, and I can pick the flavor out of any food . . . or so I thought. However, as a food science instructor, I found I needed to add more vegetarian recipes to my classes to accommodate vegetarian students. I discovered that the new tofu recipes do taste great, and they do **not** taste like soy. Soy tends to mask the flavor of other foods and make them taste bland. Add extra seasonings and spices, or marinades to ensure a full-flavored dish.

In addition to my soy aversion, I will admit that I didn't like the texture of beans. But I have now learned to enjoy them. A bean-rich chili can be an easy way to introduce beans into your diet. The chili can also be made with meat to enhance its familiarity. I add lots of frozen vegetables, everything from corn and red pepper mixture, blends of cauliflower, broccoli, and carrots, to frozen diced green peppers and onions. After cooking, everything tastes like chili. With all the different textures, you won't notice the beans (recipe in chapter 14). Some friends from Texas have assured me that sweet potatoes are also fabulous in chili. Be creative and find your own vegetable mixtures to include.

Go on a culinary adventure. Beans are an important part of the Mediterranean diet. Many finer Italian restaurants have at least one bean dish on the menu. They know how to prepare them so that they are flavorful. The seasonings, sauce, pasta and beans all complement each other for a fabulous dining experience. In my food classes, I have added Italian pasta and bean dishes which even the "bean averse" discover to be very tasty. Latin American and Caribbean dishes are often based on beans. And again, they have experience in how to season and complement the beans. The cuisine of India is largely vegetarian. Instead of choosing Americanized meat or chicken dishes, try some of the vegetarian choices, with beans providing the protein. Try Middle Eastern falafel or hummus dip which are both made from chickpeas (garbanzo beans). The Chinese were the first to domesticate soy more than 4,000 years ago. Soy is an important part of many traditional Chinese foods, and the cuisine of its neighbor, Japan. Choose traditional foods at these restaurants, rather than the Americanized versions.

You may enjoy boxed meal mixes that come with quick cooking beans. Every client to whom I have recommended these dishes really loves them. Even vegetable-hating clients find that these foods taste great, and are an easy way to introduce beans into their meals. They contain pasta, beans, and seasonings. On the back of the box are recommendations for adding other vegetables and some kind of broth, such as vegetable or chicken. You could add meat or chicken to make them more familiar. These meals are ready to eat in 15 minutes, and only take one pot to prepare. The "bean squeamish" can try a few bites of the beans, and still have lots of "regular" food to eat if they really don't like the beans.

Cater to the inner child – sneaking in vegetables.

Many children find that vegetables, especially cooked ones, taste too strong. Fortunately, as we get older, we don't taste our foods as intensely as children do. Since I counsel children as well as adults, I have learned ways to sneak vegetables into other dishes, and to recycle ideas from childhood vegetable favorites.

Some mothers become experts in tricking their kids into eating their vegetables. Maybe you can trick yourself. Why not puree some vegetables and add them to your spaghetti sauce? If you are bean-averse, you could even puree some beans. Some moms put them into hamburger or meatloaf. Sloppy Joes are everyone's childhood favorite. Add several handfuls of frozen onions and green peppers to the meat while it is browning. In my stir fry dishes I add fistfuls of broccoli slaw which become sweet when stir fried and look like noodles. Carrot cake and zucchini bread are good sources of vegetables (albeit higher calorie), and they taste great.

Remember the salads your mother used to make when you were a kid? (If you grew up in the '50s.) Rediscover the fun. How about diced vegetables floating in a gelatin mold? Carrots and raisin salad. Cole slaw with pineapple. The ever-popular three-bean salad. Tomatoes stuffed with tuna salad. And yes, tuna and chicken salad can provide another way to hide some vegetables. We all add diced celery. How about adding some finely diced red peppers, shredded carrots, and cucumbers? And while we are on the subject of '50s vegetables, the infamous green bean casserole is still everyone's favorite for Thanksgiving.

Soups are another childhood favorite that entice us to try some vegetables. Tomato soup was always my special comfort food. How about vegetable soup with or without chicken or beef? Split pea soup is a way to sneak in some legumes rich in soluble fiber. Cabbage soup is a special sweet treat. While we would like to limit cream soups, there are many types that include vegetables, and occasionally can provide some added variety to your vegetable repertoire. Don't forget vegetable broth which can be added to many other dishes. While the broth lacks the fiber of whole vegetables, it still adds phytochemicals and other vegetable nutrients. Homemade soups help keep sodium under control.

Who says carrots don't belong on a sandwich?

I love salad bars in grocery stores. They are a great place to find cut up fresh vegetables. Expand your ideas of what can go on a sandwich by experimenting with salad toppings. Tomatoes and lettuce on your sandwich are a cliché. Break out of the rut! Grated carrots, slawed red cabbage, sliced radishes make great toppings. Don't forget some sliced green, red and yellow bell peppers. Add some fresh sliced Bermuda onion for tang, or sprouts for extra crunch. Try broccoli slaw. Baby spinach or mesclun add an adult flavor to the lowly sandwich. Sliced black or green olives are special treats (and full of healthy monounsaturated fat).

How to avoid ruining the vegetables.

We all remember George Bush (the first President Bush) saying that he didn't like broccoli, and didn't want it served to him anymore. (Although why it took him until he was one year into his Presidency to work up the courage to make his wishes known, is a completely different issue.) Broccoli and other foods in the cabbage family can develop strong sulfur odors if they are over-cooked. Green beans become mushy and lose their bright green color when cooked too long. (Although there are regional and cultural differences in the degree of tenderness people prefer.) The new cuisine encourages gently cooking our vegetables. This preserves more of the heat-sensitive nutrients and preserves more of the natural sweetness of fresh produce.

To have milder tasting broccoli, and other foods in the cruciferous vegetable family such as cabbage, cauliflower and kale, choose the freshest produce. During the summer, grow your own, or go to the farmer's market to get really fresh vegetables. Older vegetables will develop more of the strong sulfur odor on cooking. If you are cooking them by boiling in water, leave the lid off. That allows the volatile sulfur compounds to evaporate into the air, instead of being trapped in the cooking water. Cook small portions in the microwave. The shorter cooking times won't cause strong flavors to develop. Steaming is another terrific way to avoid off-flavors.

Don't add baking soda to your vegetables. Although baking soda helps to preserve the bright green color of many vegetables, they make vegetables very soft and mushy, which is a turn-off to many picky eaters.

Don't add acid too early when cooking your beans. If you are cooking beans to be used in baked beans or the barbecued lentils featured in our recipe section, don't add tomato products too early in the cooking. The acid will make the beans more difficult to cook and tenderize. The overly chewy texture is sure to repel the newly reformed vegetable hater.

On the cutting edge and raw.

Raw fresh vegetables have the mildest and sweetest flavor. Either go to the salad bar, or sharpen up your knives. School lunch programs take advantage of the fact that kids will eat their carrots if they are given some ranch dressing for dipping. Any salad dressing livens up raw broccoli, carrots, celery, or cucumbers. Radishes, peppers, jicama all compete to make a crisp, cool crunch.

Dips made with non-fat sour cream remake vegetables into party favorites. My favorite is medium-hot salsa mixed into non-fat sour cream. You can alter any of your dip recipes to make them into healthy additions to your appetizer platters. Why not try some bean dip or one of the fruit-based salsas to break the monotony of vegetables with spinach dip? (Although we are not casting aspersions on this perennial favorite dip.)

You can make a salad of raw vegetables that don't fall into the ordinary category. Try zucchini, yellow squash, cucumbers or beets. You can blanch (lightly cook) a variety of colorful vegetables, such as yellow and red peppers, broccoli, and thinly sliced carrots with some cauliflower, then quick-chill and top with dressing for a still crunchy, new kind of salad.

Sweeten up the pot.

There are several easy chef-tricks for sweetening vegetables. Onions get sweet when they are "sweated," which means that they are cooked slowly over a low heat to caramelize the natural sugars. Zucchini and summer squash become delightfully sweet and flavorful when sautéed over medium heat in a tiny bit of olive oil. And jicama makes a surprisingly sweet treat when sautéed.

Roasting is another way to caramelize the sugars and bring out hidden richness in vegetables. Try roasting winter squash such as acorn or butternut at higher temperatures (450°F) to enhance the sweetness. You will find that you don't need to top with added sugar to get rich flavor. Bell peppers roasted over an open flame or heated in the oven, quickly give up their skin when wrapped in a bag for several minutes after roasting. Then slice into strips which become absolutely heavenly. You can also puree the roasted peppers for a sauce. Maybe you won't notice that you are eating vegetables and that it just happens to be good for you. Other vegetables where the flavors become fabulous when cooked at these elevated temperatures include onions, carrots, parsnips, tomatoes, oh – and best of all – sweet potatoes. It is hard to imagine that you could make them sweeter, but try roasting your sweet potatoes at 450°F for one hour. You won't need any topping, not a bit of butter. For even more suggestions on everything from broccoli to beets to artichokes, I recommend Barbara Kafka's *Roasting* (Morrow, 1995).

Salad days.

Many people find that raw vegetables are more palatable. Salads make a great vehicle for a variety of vegetables. So expand your interests beyond green stuff. Check out the sidebar to get unstuck from your normal routine. When you choose the green stuff, mix it up. Remember, darker green leaves will have more nutrients. Think about choosing romaine, spinach, watercress, red or green leaf lettuce, endive, bib or escarole. Frizze or mache are interesting French variations for your salads. Expand your color choices by adding radicchio, mesclun or red cabbage.

Again, salad bars are great for quick, healthy meals. You only buy food that you actually eat. There's no waste! When you buy head lettuce you may end up throwing out half its weight due to brown or rotting leaves. Why bother? Someone else can throw away the unusable parts, and you can pick the best parts. You can also choose lots of toppings to add a variety of vegetables, without filling your refrigerator with rotting, partially used fresh vegetables. Buy what you need for 1 - 2 days. And get extra to use on your sandwiches. If it's a really great salad bar, they will also have cut up fruit to make it easy to add fruits to your day. Pick some cantaloupe, pineapple, watermelon or strawberries. You can see what they look like without skin, and only pick the most flavorful, freshest pieces. And again, you choose plenty of variety without any waste.

Tops for Your Salad

romaine
iceberg
mesclun
watercress
red leaf
endive
bib
loose leaf
escarole
radicchio
mache
frizzé
bell peppers - red, yellow, orange, ivory, purple, and green
hot peppers
olives
cucumbers
radishes
sprouts
zucchini
yellow squash
tomatoes
onions
spinach
celery
grated carrots
red cabbage
broccoli slaw
kidney beans
green beans

Chapter 12 DASHboard

1. Many people don't like vegetables. They need some tricks to add more veggies into their diet.
2. Grow your own. Fresh vegetables are always best.
3. Beans can add variety to you r meals.
4. Sneak in the veggies.
5. Top your sandwich with cut up veggies.
6. Avoid overcooking vegetables to keep the flavor milder.
7. Raw veggies may be more appealing to people who don't like most vegetables.
8. Salad bars are great sources of cut up raw veggies. Top your salad with a variety of colorful vegetables.

Tracking my Personal DASH Diet Action Plan:

3 vegetables I will include in my diet this week:

_____

_____

1 bean dish I will try: _____

2 new salad toppers I will try: _____

_____

Chapter 13 Super Fast DASH Dining

You have made the commitment to the DASH diet. Some nights you think you just don't have the time to prepare a healthy dinner. How can you make it super easy and quick to follow? Following is a system that is boiled down to the simplest structure.

Super Simple DASH

Let's make it very simple to track your calorie level and balance the DASH diet servings for your calorie needs. Download larger copies of this form at http://dashdiet.org/forms.htm.

The next phase is super simple dinner meals. Use the check off list to see what you still need at dinnertime to complete your DASH diet plan for the entire day.

Super Fast Meals Last Minute Meals.

Start with chicken or pork chops, fresh or frozen. There is no need to thaw the frozen chicken or pork.

Cook in 375-400°F oven for 45 minutes if frozen, 35-40 minutes for fresh. You can use any kind of oven-safe pan, I use a glass pie pan. You can use a variety of toppings to make the meals interesting.

The meat should be nicely browned when done.
Choose one of the following toppings to make it
tasty:

✓ 2 T BBQ sauce during last 5 minutes of cooking.
✓ 2 T Italian dressing.
✓ Salt free seasonings: lemon pepper, Italian
  seasoning mix.
✓ 1 pat of margarine on top of chicken at beginning
  of cooking process, plus some seasonings.

Pair any of these dishes with a quick salad, either
from the salad bar or from bagged salad mixes, and
some microwaved frozen vegetables. This is super
fast, easy to pull together, and while the meal is
cooking, you have time to decompress from the day
(or better yet, get some exercise).

Another tip for making super fast healthy dinners is
to make larger portions on the weekends (for
example, using the recipes for Pile It On! Chili,
Sloppy Joes, meaty spaghetti sauce, or any of the
bean recipes), and then reheat for a quick weeknight
meal. Add a salad and frozen vegetables and you
are on track for the DASH diet.

Key: G = grain, F = fruit, V = vegetable, D = dairy, M = meat, fish, poultry, egg, N= nuts or beans, O = fats, sugars

	1200 calories	1600 calories	2000 calories	2400 calories
Breakfast	1 - 2 G 1 - 2 F 1 D	1 - 2 G 1 - 2 F 1 D 1 O	2 - 3 G 2 F 1 D 1 O	2 - 3 G 2 F 1 D 1 O
Lunch	1 - 2 G 1 - 2 V 1 - 2 D 2 oz M 1 O	1 - 3 G 1 F 1 - 2 V 1 - 2 D 2 oz M 1 O	2 - 3 G 1 F 2 V 1 - 2 D 3 oz M 1 O	2 - 3 G 1 F 2+ V 1 - 2 D 4 oz M 2 O
Snacks	0 - 1 F 0 - 1 D 0 - 1 N	0 - 1 G 0 - 1 F 0 - 1 D 0 - 1 N	0 - 1 G 0 - 1 F 0 - 1 D 0 - 1 N	1 - 2 G 0 - 1 F 1 D 0 - 1 N
Dinner	0 - 1 G 2 - 3 V 3 oz M 1 O	2 - 3 G 1 F 2 - 3 V 3 oz M 1 O	2 - 3 G 1 F 2 - 3 V 4 oz M 1 O	5 oz M 1 F 2 - 3+ V 3 - 4 G 2 O
Daily Totals G F V D M N O	(boxes)	(boxes)	(boxes)	(boxes)

✓ Shaded boxes indicate desirable extra servings of low fat or nonfat dairy and non-starchy vegetables.
✓ Circled grain boxes indicate minimum servings of whole grains.
✓ Fruit serving size is 4 oz for 1200 - 1600 calories, and 6 oz for 2000 - 2400 calories.
✓ For weight control, choose non-starchy vegetables for servings in excess of 5 per day. (Starchy vegetables include potatoes and winter squash.)
✓ If you have more than 3 dairy per day (which is a good idea), remove 1 oz meat for each extra dairy serving.

Chapter 13 DASHboard

1. Track your DASH diet servings for your calorie needs on the form in this chapter.
2. Make super fast meals that free up time to relax or exercise.
3. Use weekends to make large portions of key recipes that are rich in vegetables and beans to reheat on weeknights.

Tracking my Personal DASH Diet Action Plan:

3 super fast dinners I can prepare include: _____

_____

_____

_____

Chapter 14 - DASH Tracks, Keeping Track

How do you know if you are really getting on track with the DASH Diet Action Plan? Behavior change is more likely to be successful if you monitor your progress. All through this book you have indicated specific changes you plan to make to adopt the DASH Diet Action Plan and control your blood pressure. It is helpful to track your food intake, exercise, and weight to see how your actions pay off in terms of lowering your blood pressure. Larger copies of all of these forms are available on our web site at http://dashdiet.org/forms.htm. You will need to register as a book owner in order to access these forms and then you will be free to download them as many times as you want to continue to track your progress.

In this book we have 2 different types of forms for tracking your food intake. They are found in chapter 2 and chapter13. Choose the one that seems most useful for you. In this chapter we add forms to track exercise, weight, blood pressure, and overall health and well-being.

The blood pressure log will allow you to track how you are responding to the DASH diet. On the first line, write in your typical blood pressure readings before starting the DASH diet. Hopefully, your blood pressure will improve as you change your eating style, lose weight, and exercise. As a reminder, if your blood pressure is 140/90, 140 is the systolic reading, and 90 is the diastolic reading.

Blood Pressure Log		
Blood pressure readings	systolic (top reading)	diastolic (bottom reading)
Before starting DASH Diet		
Day 1		
Day 2		
Day 3		
Day 4		
Day 5		
Day 6		
Day 7		
Day 8		
Day 9		
Day 10		
Day 11		
Day 12		
Day 13		
Day 14		
Day 15		
Day 16		
Day 17		
Day 18		
Day 19		
Day 20		
Day 21		

For the exercise log, track the activity you

perform. Remember, set a goal of doing something active every day. If you can't do 30 or more minutes all at one time, schedule three or more 10 minute sessions.

Exercise Log			
Day	Type of Activity	Time	How do I feel?
1			
2			
3			
4			
5			
6			
7			

Getting to a healthier weight or maintaining a healthy weight is important for controlling blood pressure. The following form will provide a convenient way to keep track of your progress with weight control.

Weight Log	
Goal weight	
Initial weight	
Week 1	
Week 2	
Week 3	
Week 4	
Week 5	
Week 6	
Week 7	
Week 8	

Additional benefits of making changes in diet, weight, and activity are improved mood, higher energy level, and enhanced sense of control over your health. A diary of your feelings may provide you with additional information that will help you sustain your behavior changes. On the following page is a model for a simple diary to track how the DASH Diet Action Plan is affecting your life.

Overall DASH Diet Outcome Log	
	Mood, energy level, self-confidence, etc.
Initial	
Week 1	
Week 2	
Week 3	
Week 4	
Month 2	
Month 3	
Month 4	
Month 5	
Month 6	

Chapter 14 DASHboard

1. Track your progress.
2. Track eating.
3. Track exercise.
4. Track weight.
5. Track blood pressure.
6. Track your new attitude.

Tracking my Personal DASH Diet Action Plan:

Forms I will use to track my DASH Diet Action Plan Progress:

DASH Diet Meal Check Off ☐
DASH Diet Calorie Check Off ☐
Blood Pressure Log ☐
Exercise Log ☐
Weight Log ☐
Overall DASH Diet Outcome Log ☐

Chapter 15 The DASH Kitchen Make Over

Key to making the DASH diet work for you is setting the stage for success. And the kitchen is your stage for eating. In this chapter we will help you design a set for healthy eating, the DASH diet way.

The key DASH diet foods are fruits, vegetables, low fat and nonfat dairy, nuts and beans, lean meats, fish, and poultry. Keeping these foods on hand will make it easy to follow the diet. If, on the other hand, you keep lots of candy, chips, cookies, and ice cream in your home, you will be inclined to fill up on the wrong foods. The foods you keep on hand will determine what you eat. Keeping lots of the right foods on hand will make it easy to grab foods or make a last minute meal that will keep you on track with the DASH diet.

Let's take it step by step.

Stock up

You will want to stock your cupboards and refrigerator with staples that allow you to make a variety of meals without having to run to the store every day (unless, of course, you like to grocery shop daily). The lists that follow will provide a foundation for making it easy to DASH every day.

Making Great DASH Choices

It is easy to make great choices by buying whole grains, fruits and vegetables. But what about dairy and meats, fish, and poultry?

Key to a heart healthy diet is choosing foods that are low in saturated fats. In the dairy group, the absolute best choice is nonfat (skim) milk. It has all the calcium, protein, and none of the saturated fats that are found in whole milk and most other dairy foods. If you are lactose intolerant, you can find lactose-free milk or take lactose-digesting enzymes to ease digestion. Another option is low carb milk (technically a dairy beverage, not milk), which has the added benefit of extra calcium, extra protein, and extra rich taste compared with regular nonfat milk.

Nonfat yogurt is equally good. If you are watching calories, choose yogurts with little or no added sugars. The labels on yogurt can be confusing, because of the milk sugar which was in the original milk. (And for carb counters, almost all of the milk sugar has been converted to lactic acid in yogurts. The actual sugar content is minimal.) Choose yogurts with less than 120 calories for 8 ounce servings, or less than 100 calories for 6 ounce servings. As an added benefit, most people with lactose intolerance can handle yogurt very well.

When choosing cheese, buy reduced fat or nonfat cheese for home. When you are dining out, you generally don't have a low fat cheese option available, so make sure your home is stocked with reduced fat cheese. Cheese is one of the highest sources of saturated fat in the typical American diet. Cheeses are very low in lactose.

Which is better, butter or margarine. A soft margarine, which doesn't contain trans fats is your best choice. For special baking or cooking, you can occasionally use butter, as long as you use it rarely. I choose butter for special meals for its flavor, but I rarely use either margarine or butter as part of my routine diet.

Meats and poultry are other common sources of saturated fats. In general, choosing select grades of beef, and cuts with the words "round" or "loin" in their names will give you lean cuts. Appendix A provides you with a list of beef, pork, and poultry cuts and their calorie and fat contents. And of course, skinless chicken and turkey are low in saturated fat.

Most fish and seafood is very low in saturated fat. While shrimp may be high in cholesterol, it is still considered to be a good choice as part of a heart healthy diet since it is very low in fat. (As long as it is not fried or swimming in butter.) Most fatty fish contain special omega-3 fatty acids that are considered to be very heart healthy. Even the fattiest fish are still in the lean range when compared with meat and poultry.

Coconut oil is a surprising source of saturated fat. This may be found in popcorn, especially commercially prepared fresh popcorn.

Trans fats are found in many baked goods, such

as pastries, snack crackers, and pie crusts. The newer food labels will contain trans fat content so that you can choose to limit these foods. You can limit trans fats by avoiding foods with hydrogenated or partially hydrogenated fats.

Staples

Canned/bottled/dry
diced tomatoes, no added salt
tomato sauce, no added salt
tomato paste, no added salt
kidney beans, no added salt
black beans, no added salt
lentils
tuna, canned in water, low salt
canned salmon, low salt
canned chicken, low salt
extra virgin olive oil
canola oil
vegetable oil
white and/or yellow corn meal
oatmeal
cereals without added sugar, and high in fiber
various types of pasta: rotini, spaghetti, angel hair, shells, linguine, whole grain, etc.
nuts, unsalted

Spices and herbs
bag of onions
bulbs of garlic
shallots
dry spices including basil, oregano, parsley flakes, thyme, marjoram, paprika, rosemary, ginger, poultry seasoning, sage, onion powder, garlic powder, etc.
taco sauce or seasonings
chili mix
salt substitutes, including lemon-pepper
reduced sodium soy sauce
stir fry sauces/mixes, low sodium
potato seasoning mixes
Worcestershire sauce

Frozen
individual and mixed vegetables
sliced pepper and onion mix
diced onions
diced green peppers
frozen skinless boneless chicken breasts
frozen 95% lean ground sirloin (& patties)
pizza crusts
corn or flour tortillas
whole wheat pita
frozen yogurt, with no added sugar
frozen fruit

Refrigerated
lemon juice
lime juice
dark green lettuces
baby carrots
grape tomatoes
grated carrots
sliced carrots
cole slaw mix

broccoli slaw
salad dressings
sliced deli meats, low
sodium
barbecue sauce, low
sodium
whole wheat bread
oatmeal bran bread
ketchup

Fresh From the Market

Fresh Additions
salad bar for cut up fresh
    items:
lettuce
radishes
peppers
onions
carrots
broccoli
cauliflower
red cabbage
cucumber
beets
fresh fruit

Produce Counter
fresh fruits, vegetables,
greens, fresh herbs

Meat Counter
fresh fish
lean meat, poultry
(see Appendix A)

Dairy
low fat or nonfat cheeses
    - cheddar, Swiss,
    colby/jack, Parmesan,
    Romano, mozzarella,
    sliced and grated
    cheeses
light individually
    packaged cheeses
    such as Baby Bel™,
    Laughing Cow™,
    string cheese, Kraft
    2% Singles™, 2% or
    1% cottage cheese
nonfat yogurt, artificially
    sweetened
skim milk or low carb
    skim milk
egg substitutes
eggs

Equipment

Having the right equipment on hand will make your life easier, whether you like to cook or don't want to spend your time cooking.

✓ George Foreman® Grill or other similar countertop grill. This allows the quick preparation of lean meats, fish, and poultry. The newer versions have removable grill surfaces for easy cleanup.

✓ Toaster oven - great for making small meals or reheating certain leftovers

✓ Microwave - always great for reheating or making quick scrambled eggs

✓ Blenders - can help with pureeing vegetables to sneak into sauces or soups, in addition to making great smoothies.

✓ Digital kitchen scale - helps to make it easy to avoid "portion distortion."

✓ Food processors - make it a breeze to cut up vegetables.

✓ Mandoline or V-Slicers - even faster cut up veggies.

✓ Instant read digital thermometers - tell you when your meat is cooked correctly, and when your leftovers are heated enough (165° F).

✓ Great super sharp knives, not serrated - make cutting up vegetables easier. Thinner blades are easier to push through larger vegetables.

Cookbooks, recipes

Some cookbooks which are supportive of the DASH diet include the following.

Quick and Easy

For the person who likes convenience and needs ideas

that are fast, but still wonderful
- ✓ Cooking Light's 5 Ingredient, 15 Minute Cookbook by Anne Chappell Cain, Oxford House, 1999.
- ✓ Cooking Light One-Dish Meals Cookbook by Susan McIntosh, Oxford House.
- ✓ Lickety Split Meals by Zonya Foco, ZHI Publishing, 1998.
- ✓ Quick & Healthy, Low-Fat, Carb Conscious Cooking, by Brenda J. Ponichtera, ScaleDown Publishing, Inc., 2004

Absolute must-have
- ✓ Better Homes and Garden New Cook Book, 12th Edition, Meredith Books, 2002. (Older versions of this cookbook are also fabulous.)

For the serious cook
Anything by Julia Child, including,
- ✓ The Way to Cook, Julia Child, Knopf, 1989.
- ✓ Roasting. A Simple Art, Barbara Kafka, William Morrow and Company, Inc. 1995.
- ✓ Le Cordon Bleu Complete Cooking Techniques, Jeni Wright & Eric Treuille, Cassell plc, 1996.

Web sites for DASH-friendly recipes

Find recipes for lean beef and pork
http://www.beefitswhatsfordinner.com
http://www.porkandhealth.com

Low fat and nonfat dairy recipes
http://3aday.org/recipes/index.html
http://www.ilovecheese.com/recipes.asp

Add more fruits and vegetables to your diet
http://5aday.org/html/recipes/onthemenu.php

Include nuts, beans, and soy.
http://www.almondsarein.com/recipes/
http://www.michiganbean.org/cooking.html
http://www.pea-lentil.com/recipes/
http://www.walnuts.org/recipes/rcp_index.shtml
http://www.talksoy.com/Recipes/default.htm
http://www.soyfoods.com/recipes/

For more web sites (or if these sites have changed
and aren't working), see
http://dashdiet.org/links.htm

Chapter 15 DASHboard

1. Stock up on DASH foods.
2. Refrigerator: 2% or low fat cheeses, fresh veggies from the salad bar, bagged cut up vegetables, fresh fruits, lean meats, fish, poultry, low fat or nonfat milk or yogurt.
3. Freezer: frozen vegetables, frozen fruits, 95% extra lean ground sirloin and patties, boneless and skinless chicken breasts, diced peppers and onions.
4. Cupboards: seasonings, canned no-salt beans, no added salt tomato products, including sauce, diced, and whole tomatoes. Sugar substitutes.
5. Equipment: countertop grills, food processors, great knives, microwave, blenders, instant read thermometers.
6. Great cookbooks provide lots of ideas for your DASH diet meals.
7. More recipes can be found at the web sites listed at the end of the chapter.

Tracking my Personal DASH Diet Action Plan:

Items I plan to add to my kitchen include:

_____

_____

_____

Chapter 16 Fabulous Recipes for the DASH to Success

Ground Beef (Extra-lean) Recipes

"Pile it On!" Chili

So named because it tastes great and it piles on vegetables. This chili is very low in calories because of all the vegetables. You will get full before you can overdo this great tasting chili. Top with shredded light cheese and baked tortilla strips if desired.

1 pound ground sirloin, 95% extra-lean
1/2 bag frozen onion, peppers combo
2 - 3 garlic cloves, minced or squeezed through a
    garlic press
1 medium can diced tomatoes, no added salt
1 medium can tomato sauce, no added salt
1 can kidney beans
1 can black beans
2 tablespoon chili powder
2 tablespoon paprika
1/2 bag frozen mixed broccoli, cauliflower, and
carrots
1 cup frozen corn

Heat a large nonstick skillet over medium-high heat. Add ground beef (you can substitute ground turkey breast if desired), cook 3 minutes, turn heat down to medium. Add peppers, onions and garlic. (High temperatures make garlic turn bitter and brown.) Continue cooking about 5 more minutes, or until thoroughly browned and onions are soft.

Add tomatoes, beans and seasonings. Mix well, allow to simmer about 5 minutes. Then add mixed vegetables and corn.

Simmer 30 - 60 minutes. If the chili starts getting really thick, you could add water or more tomato sauce.

Yield 12, 1- cup servings. Nutrition DASHboard: 204 calories, 13 g protein, 24 g carbohydrates, 7 g fat, 26 mg cholesterol, 7 g fiber, 379 mg sodium, 583 mg potassium.

Alternatives: If you prefer, you can use fresh diced onions, and red, green, and yellow pepper strips. You can add any other vegetables that you think would be interesting. Friends from Texas tell me that sweet potato chunks are wonderful in chili.

Baked Tortilla Strips

Cut 2 corn tortillas into 1/2-inch strips. Place on tray in oven or toaster oven. Heat at 400°F for 5 minutes, or until lightly browned. Use to garnish the chili.

Sloppy Joes

1 pound extra-lean ground beef, 95% lean
1 cup chopped onions, fresh or frozen
1 cup chopped green peppers, fresh or frozen
2 garlic cloves, minced or squeezed through a garlic press
14.5-oz can tomato sauce, no salt added
2 tablespoons red wine vinegar
1 teaspoon paprika
2 teaspoons Worcestershire sauce
1/2 teaspoon chili powder
1/2 teaspoon black pepper
dash (or more) hot pepper sauce or cayenne pepper

Heat a large nonstick skillet over medium-high heat. Add ground beef, cook 3 minutes, turn heat down to medium. Add peppers, onions, and garlic. (High temperatures make garlic turn bitter and brown.) Continue cooking 5 or more minutes, or until thoroughly browned.
Add tomato sauce and all other ingredients. Reduce heat and simmer 10 - 15 minutes.

Yield 5 servings. Nutrient DASHboard: 224 calories, 27 g protein, 13 g carbohydrates, 7 g fat, 76 mg cholesterol, 2 g fiber, 114 mg sodium, 798 mg potassium.

Extra Lean Meaty Spaghetti Sauce

1 pound extra-lean ground beef, 95% lean
2 garlic cloves, minced or squeezed through garlic press
1/2 cup chopped onions, fresh or frozen
14.5 oz can tomato sauce, no salt added
14.5 oz can diced tomatoes, no salt added
1 teaspoon Italian seasoning
1 teaspoon dried basil

Heat a large nonstick skillet over medium-high heat. Add ground beef, cook 3 minutes, turn heat down to medium. Add onions and garlic. Continue cooking about 5 more minutes, or until thoroughly browned. (High temperatures make garlic turn bitter and brown.)
Add diced tomatoes and tomato sauce. Simmer 10 - 15 minutes. Add seasonings in last few minutes of cooking.

Yield 6 servings. Nutrition DASHboard: 184 calories, 24 g protein, 8 g carbohydrates, 6 g fat, 67 mg cholesterol, 2 g fiber, 105 mg sodium, 733 mg potassium.

Extra Lean Beef Taco Filling

1 pound extra lean ground sirloin, 95% lean
1/2 bottle mild or medium taco sauce
1 cup diced onions, fresh or frozen
1 cup diced green peppers, fresh or frozen

Heat a large nonstick skillet over medium-high heat.
Add ground beef, cook 3 minutes, turn heat down to
medium. Add onions and peppers. Continue
cooking 5 or more minutes, or until thoroughly
browned.
Add taco sauce, reduce heat and simmer 5 - 10
minutes.

Yield 4 servings (enough for 3 medium sized tacos
for each). Nutrition DASHboard:

Chicken Dishes

Low Sodium Chicken Piccata

1 pound chicken breasts, boneless, skinless (4 half
    breasts)
1/2 cup yellow cornmeal
1 teaspoon lemon-pepper seasoning mix
1 cup low sodium chicken broth
1 tablespoon olive oil
2 tablespoon lemon juice
2 tablespoon butter

Preheat chicken broth over medium heat.

Place each chicken breast half on a sheet of plastic wrap. Sprinkle with water, then place another sheet of plastic wrap on top. (The water keeps the wrap from sticking together and makes it easier to peel apart.) Pound chicken to about 1/4 inch thickness using a mallet or rolling pin.

Mix cornmeal and pepper on a plate or pie pan. Drag chicken through cornmeal mix, coating both sides well.

Heat oil in a large nonstick skillet over medium-high heat. (If the oil is smoking the temperature is too high.) Add chicken and cook 4 minutes on each side or until browned. Remove chicken from pan, place on plate with cover (pot lid or bowl), to keep warm. Add lemon juice and hot chicken broth to skillet, scraping pan to loosen browned bits. Reduce heat to medium, stir in butter. Return chicken to pan, cook 3 minutes or until done (internal temperature 165°F). Remove from heat, serve immediately.

Yield 4. Nutrition DASHboard: 287 calories, 28 g protein, 20 g carbohydrate, 12 g fat, 82 mg cholesterol, 94 mg sodium, 299 mg potassium.

Recipe adapted from Sara Moulton Cooks at Home

Carribean Chicken

1 pound chicken breasts, boneless, skinless (4 half-
    breasts)
1 teaspoon salt
dash pepper
dash onion powder
dash garlic powder
dash cayenne pepper
dash paprika
1 tablespoon vegetable oil
1 13-1/4 oz can pineapple chunks
1 teaspoon ginger
2 oranges, one for juice and peel, one for peeled
    orange slices
1/4 cup honey
2 teaspoon flour
2 tablespoon water
1 orange, peeled, sliced

Season chicken with salt, pepper, onion powder,
garlic powder, paprika, cayenne pepper. Sauté in
hot oil until well browned on all sides. Drain excess
fat.
Drain pineapple, and reserve juice for sauce.
Combine pineapple juice, ginger, 2 teaspoon orange
peel, ⅓ cup orange juice (squeezed from orange)
and honey. Pour over chicken. Cover and simmer 40
minutes or until tender.
Remove chicken to a warm serving platter.
Mix flour and water together until smooth. Stir into
pan drippings, and heat to boiling while stirring.
Add pineapple chunks and orange slices from
second orange (remove peel). Heat just until fruit is

warm, serve over chicken.

Yield 6. Nutrition DASHboard: 295 calories, 27 g protein, 36 g carbohydrates, 5 g fat, 66 mg cholesterol, 2 mg fiber, 83 mg sodium, 371 mg potassium.

Chicken Cacciatore
1 1/2 pound boneless, skinless chicken breasts
1 can (16 oz.) stewed tomatoes, no added salt
1 package frozen sliced onion and pepper combo
1 teaspoon Italian herb seasoning
1 can (14.5 oz.) tomato sauce, no added salt
1/4 teaspoon red pepper flakes

Spray a large saucepan with non-stick coating. Add chicken and remaining ingredients.
Cover and simmer, stirring occasionally, for 25-35 minutes.

Yield 4 servings. Nutrition DASHboard 185 calories, 28 g protein, 14 g carbohydrate, 2 g fat, 66 mg cholesterol, 3 g fiber, 122 mg sodium, 808 mg potassium.

Alternatively, this recipe could be prepared in a slow cooker. If you are having potatoes with the meal, slice them, and place them underneath the chicken.

Pollo Alla Griglio

This is a grilled chicken, pan-finished with lemon sauce, placed on top of baby greens, with roasted potatoes. You could also substitute chicken piccata for the grilled chicken.

1 pound chicken breast, skinless boneless
1 tablespoon olive oil
1 garlic clove
1 cup low sodium chicken broth
2 tablespoon lemon juice
1/4 teaspoon ground black pepper
2 tablespoon butter
1/2 teaspoon poultry seasoning
4 medium red potatoes, quartered
1 tablespoon olive oil
nonstick cooking spray
baby greens
20 grape tomatoes

Preheat oven to 400 °F. Quarter potatoes, place in small roasting pan, drizzle with olive oil or spray with nonstick cooking spray. Roasting in 400 °F oven for 30 minutes.
Heat chicken broth over medium heat.
Rub chicken breasts with cut garlic clove, and sprinkle with mixed sage and rosemary. Spray chicken with nonstick cooking spray and place on hot grill. Cook 4 minutes on each side, or until browned. Place grilled chicken on plate and cover with pot lid or aluminum foil.
Heat 1 tablespoon olive oil in large, nonstick skillet over medium heat. Add warm chicken broth, lemon juice, ground pepper, and butter. Place grilled chicken and roasted potatoes in sauce, and heat 3 - 4

minutes, turning to coat with sauce.
Place on top of baby greens and grape tomatos.

Yield 4 servings. Nutrition DASHboard: 349 calories,
30 g protein, 23 g carbohydrate, 15 g fat, 83 mg
cholesterol, 152 mg sodium, 866 mg potassium.

Roasted Chicken with Potatoes, Carrots, and Brussels Sprouts

1 whole chicken, about 5 pounds
4 medium potatoes, with skin, cut into large chunks
2 cup Brussels sprouts
2 cup carrots, sliced into 1" sections
1 tablespoon olive oil

Preheat oven to 350 °F. Place washed and dried
chicken in roasting pan. Dust with poultry
seasonings, inside and out.
Place cut up potatoes, sliced carrots, and Brussels
sprouts around chicken, drizzle with olive oil. Add 1
cup water to bottom of pan (or white wine or low
sodium chicken broth)
Roast in 350°F oven for 60 minutes.

Yield 4 servings. Nutrition DASHboard: 319 calories,
32 g protein, 42 g carbohydrates, 3 g fat, 66 mg
cholesterol, 7 g fiber, 142 mg sodium, 1465 mg
potassium.

Alternately you could use a frozen mixture of
carrots, cauliflower, and broccoli.

Pepper-Slaw Chicken Stirfry

1 pound boneless, skinless chicken breasts, cut into 1/2"
x 2" strips
1/2 bag broccoli slaw
1/2 bag frozen onion and pepper mixture (or for less
soft texture, use sliced fresh onions and red, orange,
yellow and green peppers)
low sodium stir fry sauce
2 tablespoon peanut oil or canola oil

Heat large skillet over medium-high heat. Add peanut
(or canola) oil.
When oil is hot (but not smoking), add 1/2 of chicken
strips to oil, and sauté 1 - 2 minutes, stirring with wooden
spatula until cooked on all sides.
Remove chicken, place on warm plate, repeat with rest of
chicken. Cover plate with all chicken to keep warm.
Add pepper and onion mixture to pan. Stirfry 3 - 4
minutes. (Watch out for splatters from the moisture if
you use frozen vegetables.) Add broccoli slaw, and
sauté until tender.
Add 1/4 cup stir fry sauce, and add chicken back into
pan. Stir well to reheat chicken and to mix sauce.

Yield 4 (2 cup) servings. Nutrition DASHboard:

Alternate recipe: Chinese Vegetable Stir Fry. Same basic
recipe as above, substituting for the vegetables:
chopped bok choy, water chestnuts, sliced mushrooms,
and bean sprouts. You can find frozen stirfry mixtures
that will also work well. Be careful of splatters when
adding frozen vegetables to hot oil.

Pork recipes

Peach-Mustard Glazed Pork Chops

4 (4 oz) boneless pork loin chops, 3/4 inch thick
   (trim all visible fat)
1 (16oz can) peach slices in extra light syrup,
undrained
2 tablespoon peach preserves
2 tablespoon Dijon mustard
1 teaspoon Worcestershire sauce
1 teaspoon black pepper

Combine peaches, preserves, mustard and
Worcestershire sauce in medium bowl.
Heat large nonstick skillet over medium-high heat
until hot.
Season chops with pepper. Add chops to skillet;
brown on both sides.
Add peach mixture to skillet; reduce heat to low.
Cover; cook 5 minutes. Serve pork chops topped
with peach mixture. Garnish with fresh raspberries,
if desired.

Yield 4 servings. Nutrition DASHboard: 236 calories,
22 g protein, 15 g carbohydrate, 10 g fat, 73 mg
cholesterol, 96 mg sodium, 458 mg potassium.
Recipe from National Pork Producers Council.

Bean recipes

Beans are not a common part of the typical American diet. The following recipes were developed or modified with my students at the University of Illinois at Chicago, in the introductory foods class. All of the recipes were favorites. Since college students are notoriously picky, you can be sure that these very appetizing recipes will help you expand your own repertoire of bean dishes.

Rice with Black-Eyed Peas & Tomatoes

1 tablespoon olive oil
1 large onion, peeled and finely chopped
1 garlic clove, peeled and finely chopped, squeezed
    through a garlic press
1 1/2 cups long-grain white rice
16-oz can black-eyed peas, undrained
28-oz can diced tomatoes, drained
11/2 tablespoon chili powder
1/2 teaspoon cumin
1 teaspoon crushed dried oregano
1/4 teaspoon cayenne pepper
3 cup water
dash salt, pepper

Add olive oil to nonstick skillet, over medium heat. When oil is hot, add onion and sauté until translucent, about 5 minutes. Reducing the heat to prevent browning, and add garlic and continue to saute until lightly browned. (Do not cook the garlic at too high a heat or allow to turn dark, since it will turn bitter.)

Put the sautéed onions and garlic into a large pot, add the remaining ingredients, and bring to a boil over medium high heat, stirring occasionally.

Reduce the heat and simmer, partially covered, until the rice is tender, about 30 minutes, stirring occasionally to ensure that everything is evenly distributed.

Season with pepper to taste.

Yield 8 (1 cup) servings. Nutrition DASHboard: 230 calories, 5 g protein, 47 g carbohydrates, 2 g fat, 6 g fiber, 61 mg sodium, 568 mg potassium.

Lentil Confetti Salad

1 cup lentils, rinsed
3 cup water
1 cup rice, cooked and warm
1/2 cup light Italian dressing
1 large tomato, seeded and diced
1/2 cup finely diced red onion
1/2 cup celery, chopped
1/4 cup pimento stuffed olives, sliced
1/4 cup sweet green pepper, medium diced
1 tablespoon fresh parsley, chopped

In a saucepan, pour water over lentils, bring to a boil, and simmer 20 minutes or until lentils are tender.

Separately, cook rice per package directions.

Combine drained lentils with rice and all vegetables. Toss lightly with dressing.

Yield 8 servings. Nutrition DASHboard: 131 calories, 8 g protein, 22 g carbohydrates, 2 g fat, 8 g fiber, 99 g sodium, 321 mg potassium.

Recipe adapted from USA Dry Pea & Lentil Council

Black Beans with Tomatoes and Cilantro*

This is a wonderful, healthy dip for baked corn tortillas (whole grain) or for cut up pepper strips.

15- oz can black beans, drained and rinsed
1 1/2 tablespoon peanut or corn oil
1 medium onion, chopped
1 teaspoon garlic, chopped
14 oz can diced tomatoes, drained
1/2 teaspoon Tabasco sauce
1/2 teaspoon salt
2 tablespoons fresh cilantro, chopped

Heat oil in a small skillet over medium high-heat; add the onions and garlic. Sauté stirring until onion is almost translucent but still firm, about 2 minutes. Add tomatoes and cook, Stirring frequently, for 2 minutes more.
Add black beans, Tabasco, and salt. Stir to combine. Cover skillet. Cook until beans are heated through about 2 minutes.

Remove from heat. Stir in 1 tablespoon of cilantro.
Transfer to serving dish and sprinkle with
remaining cilantro. Serve immediately.

Yield 8 (1/2 cup) servings. Nutrition DASHboard:
110 calories, 5 g protein, 17 g carbohydrates, 3 g fat,
6 g fiber, 23 mg sodium, 333 mg potassium.

Pasta e Fagioli alla Venezia*

1 can kidney beans
1/4 cup olive oil
1 cup onion, chopped coarse
1 cup carrot, chopped coarse
1 celery stalk with leaves, chopped coarse
1 tablespoon garlic, chopped fine
3 tablespoon fresh basil, chopped fine, or 1 teaspoon
    dried basil
1 cup canned Italian plum tomatoes, chopped
1 teaspoon dried rosemary, crushed
1/4 teaspoon red pepper flakes
1/4 teaspoon dried sage
2 cup chicken or vegetable broth, or boiling water
2 cup dried whole grain pasta

Heat oil in large heavy saucepan over medium high
heat. Add onions and sauté until they begin to turn
golden. Add carrot, celery, and garlic.
Cook for a few minutes more, stirring occasionally.
Add beans, tomatoes, rosemary, sage , red pepper
flakes, and 1 cup boiling liquid. Turn heat to high

and bring to boil. Reduce heat to simmer. Cook covered, until beans are tender, about 15 minutes. Transfer about 2 ladles of beans and their liquid to food processor, blender, or food mill. Process to a thick puree and stir back into soup.

About 15 minutes before serving, bring soup to a boil and add pasta and the remaining cup of broth. Stir occasionally until pasta is cooked *al dente*, about 8 to 10 minutes.

Remove from heat and stir in pepper to taste. Ladle into soup bowls and sprinkle each serving with Parmesan cheese.

Yield 6 servings. Nutrition DASHboard: 167 calories, 8 g protein, 33 g carbohydrates, 1.5 g fat, 7 g fiber, 498 mg sodium, 613 mg potassium.

* Recipes adapted from Michigan Bean Commission

Miscellaneous Recipes

Southwestern Egg White Omelette

1/2 cup egg substitutes or 4 egg whites
1/4 cup diced red bell pepper
1 tablespoon diced jalapeño peppers (if desired)
1/4 cup diced onions

Heat nonstick omelette pan or small skillet, over
medium heat. Spray with nonstick cooking spray.
Sauté peppers and onions until slightly soft.
Pour 1/2 cup egg substitute or egg whites over
onion pepper mixture. Gently lift sides of omelette,
as egg begins to set, to allow uncooked egg to slide
underneath and firm up. Repeat until top of
omelette is relatively set. Flip once. Allow to cook
for a few seconds, then fold over, and slip onto
plate.

Yield 1 serving. Nutrition DASHboard: 90 calories,
13 g protein, 9 g carbohydrates, 0 g fat, 0 mg
cholesterol, 2 g fiber, 232 mg sodium, 329 mg
potassium.

Alternately, you could use 1/4 cup diced tomato,
1/4 green peppers, and a few sliced mushrooms.

Parmesan Roasted Red Potatoes

1 pound new (small) red potatoes
1/2 cup freshly grated Parmesan cheese
non-stick cooking spray
1 teaspoon dried oregano
1 teaspoon dried basil

Preheat oven to 400 °F. In small roasting pan place red potatoes. Spray with nonstick cooking spray. Sprinkle with Parmesan cheese, oregano, and basil. Cook about 40 minutes, or until tender.

Yield 4 servings. Nutrition DASHboard: 164 calories, 6 g protein, 21 g carbohydrates, 1 g fat, 9 mg cholesterol, 2 g fiber, 159 mg sodium, 493 mg potassium.

Low Fat, Low Salt Tuna Salad

6 oz very low sodium tuna
2 tablespoon low fat mayonnaise
1/4 cup diced celery
1/4 cup diced red peppers
dash ground pepper

Mix all ingredients together. If you want more color and crunch, you could also add some grated carrots. A diced egg could add some more protein and additional creaminess (although it would significantly increase cholesterol).

Yield 2 servings. Nutrition DASHboard: 142 calories, 21 g protein, 1.5 g carbohydrate, 6 g fat, 50 mg cholesterol, 267 mg sodium, 205 mg potassium.

Chicken Waldorf Salad

6 oz chicken meat
1/4 c diced celery
1/4 c diced apple
2 T coarsely chopped walnuts
1/4 cup light mayonnaise
1 t lemon juice

Toss chicken, celery, apples, and nuts together lightly. Chill.
Mix salad dressing and lemon juice. Gently stir into chicken mixture. Chill.

Yield 4 (1/2 cup) servings. Nutrition DASHboard: 137 calories, 13 g protein, 4 g carbohydrates, 41 mg cholesterol, 114 mg sodium, 160 mg potassium.

Alternately, for Tuna Waldorf Salad, substitute a can of low sodium tuna for the chicken.

Italian Cole Slaw

1 1/4 cup shredded cabbage   *2 pkg splenda*
⅓ cup shredded carrots   *peppar*
⅓ cup green or red bell pepper, sliced
2 tablespoons sliced red onions
2 tablespoons olive oil
3 T red wine vinegar
1/4 teaspoon celery seeds

Mix all ingredients. Chill.

Yield 6 (1/2 cup) servings. Nutrition DASHboard: 63 calories, 7 g carbohydrates, 4 g fat, 1 g fiber, 16 mg sodium, 153 mg potassium.

Halibut in Balsamic Reduction

1 pound halibut
1 teaspoon olive oil
1 shallot, minced
⅓ cup balsamic vinegar
1/2 cup chicken broth, warm

Preheat oven to 450°F. Cut halibut into 4 pieces.
Place halibut on baking sheet which has been
sprayed with nonstick cooking spray, spray again.
Bake in oven 6 - 8 minutes, depending on thickness.
Heat chicken broth for 1 minute in microwave on
high.
In small skillet or saute pan, over medium heat, heat
1 T olive oil. Add minced shallot, cook until
translucent and soft. Add balsamic vinegar and
warm chicken broth. Continue to cook over
medium-high heat until volume is reduced by half.
Spoon balsamic reduction over halibut.

Yield 4 servings. Nutrition DASHboard: 169 calories,
24 g protein, 7 g carbohydrates, 4 g fat, 37 mg
cholesterol, 83 mg sodium, 532 mg potassium.

Smashed red potatoes

2 pounds red potatoes, cut into large chunks
4 - 8 oz skim milk (warm)
1/4 teaspoon ground black pepper
1 tablespoon butter, soft or melted

Cut potatoes (do not peel) into large chunks, 1 1/2 - 2". Cook 20-25 minutes in boiling water until very tender. When the potatoes are done, drain, and put back in pan to allow excess moisture to evaporate. Add butter, pepper, and skim milk according to the desired consistency. Mash gently, leaving skins relatively intact.

Yield 6. Nutrition DASHboard: 145 calories, 4 g protein, 28 g carbohydrate, 2 g fat, 6 mg cholesterol, 2 g fiber, 31 mg sodium, 652 mg potassium.

Oven Potato Fries

4 medium baking potatoes (about 1 1/2 - 2 pounds)
salt-free seasoning mix (or 1/2 teaspoon pepper, 1
    teaspoon paprika, 1/2 teaspoon onion powder,
    1/2 teaspoon garlic powder)
1 tablespoon vegetable oil
nonstick cooking spray

Preheat oven to 450 °F.
Slice potatoes into wedges, with a maximum width

of 1/2 inch. Place potato slices, oil, and seasonings into a plastic zipper bag. Shake well to distribute seasonings on potato surfaces.

Spray baking sheet with nonstick cooking spray. Arrange potato slices on baking sheet. (To minimize clean up, you can line baking sheet first with aluminum foil.)

Bake at 450°F for 30 - 35 minutes, or until golden brown.

Yield 6 servings. Nutrition DASHboard: 147 calories, 3.5 g protein, 29 g carbohydrates, 2.5 g fat, 0 mg cholesterol, 3 g fiber, 14 mg sodium, 732 mg potassium.

Appendix A Calories and Fat for Meat and Poultry

Calories and Fat for 3 oz Cooked Lean Beef

	Calories	Fat g	Saturated fats g	Cholesterol mg
Top round roast, broiled	153	4.2	1.4	71
Eye Round, roasted	143	4.2	1.5	59
Shoulder pot roast, roasted	136	4.7	1.6	54
Round tip roast, roasted	147	5.7	1.8	60
Shoulder steak, braised	161	6.0	1.9	80
Top sirloin steak, broiled	166	6.1	2.4	76
Bottom round, roasted	161	6.3	2.1	66
Top loin steak, broiled	176	8.0	3.1	65
Tenderloin steak, broiled	175	8.1	3.0	71
T-bone steak, broiled	172	8.2	3.0	48
Tri-tip roast, roasted	177	8.2	3.0	70
NY strip steak, broiled				
Ground beef, 95% lean, pan-broiled	139	5.0	2.2	65
Ground beef, 90% lean, pan-broiled	173	9.1	3.7	70
Ground beef, 85% lean, pan-broiled	197	11.9	4.7	73

Calories and Fat for 3 oz Cooked Lean Pork

	Calories	Fat g	Saturated fats g	Cholesterol mg
Pork tenderloin, roasted	140	4	1	65
Pork top loin roast, roasted	170	6	2	65
Pork top loin chop, broiled	170	7	2	70
Pork loin center chop, broiled	170	7	3	70
Pork sirloin roast, roasted	180	9	3	75
Ham, lean, roasted	145	5.5	1.8	53

Calories and Fat for 3 oz Cooked Lean Poultry

	Calories	Fat g	Saturated fats g	Cholesterol mg
Chicken breast, with skin, roasted	167	6.6	1.9	71
Chicken Breast, skinless, roasted	140	3.0	0.9	72
Chicken thigh, with skin, roasted	210	13.2	3.7	7.9
Chicken thigh, skinless, roasted	178	9.2	2.6	81
Turkey breast, skinless, roasted	115	0.6	0.2	71
Turkey whole, with skin, roasted	146	4.9	1.4	89
Ground turkey, cooked	200	11.2	2.9	87
Ground turkey breast, cooked	98	3.8	1.0	44

Calories and Fat for 3 oz Cooked Fish and Seafood

	Calories	Fat g	Saturated fats g	Cholesterol mg
Blue crab	100	1	0	90
Catfish	140	9	2	50
Clams (about 12 small)	100	1.5	0	55
Cod	90	0.5	0	45
Flounder/sole	100	1.5	0.5	60
Haddock	100	1	0	80
Halibut	110	2	0	35
Lobster	80	0	0	60
Mackerel	210	13	1.5	60
Ocean perch	110	2	0	50
Orange roughy	80	1	0	20
Oysters, about 12 medium	100	3.5	1	115
Pollock	90	1	0	80
Rainbow trout	140	6	2	60
Rockfish	100	2	0	40
Salmon, Atlantic/Coho	160	7	1	50
Salmon, Chum/Pink	130	4	1	70
Salmon, Sockeye	180	9	1.5	75
Scallops, 6 large, 14 small	120	1	0	55
Shrimp	80	1	0	165
Swordfish	130	4.5	1	40
Tuna, canned in water	116	0.8	0.2	30
White fish	172	7.5	1.2	77

Appendix B. Omega-3 fatty acid content for fish and seafood

Food Item	EPA (grams)	DHA (grams)
Cod liver oil (1 Tablespoon)	1.0	1.5
Mackerel (3.5 ounces)	0.9	1.4
Salmon (3.5 ounces)	0.8	0.6
Herring (3.5 ounces)	0.7	0.9
Anchovy (3.5 ounces)	0.5	0.9
Tuna (3.5 ounces)	0.3	0.9
Blue fish (3.5 ounces)	0.2	0.5
Swordfish (3.5 ounces)	0.1	0.5
EPA - eicosapentaenoic acid, DHA - docosahexenoic acid		

Appendix C Serving Sizes

Serving Sizes	
Grains The serving sizes are designed to be about 1 ounce dry weight and about 80 calories. Watch cereal serving sizes which can range from 1/4 cup to 11/2 cup.	1 slice bread 1/2 cup cooked pasta, rice, cereal, corn 1 oz dry cereal 1/4 bagel 1/2 English muffin or hamburger or hot dog bun 2 cups popcorn 2 small cookies
Fruits	6 oz juice (4 oz for 1200 or 1600 calorie diets) medium fruit 1/4 cup dried fruit 1/2 cup canned fruit 1 cup large diced raw fruit
Vegetables	1/2 cup cooked vegetables 1 cup leafy greens 6 oz vegetable juice
Dairy	8 oz skim or low fat milk 8 oz low fat/fat-free yogurt 1oz reduced fat cheese 1/2 cup fat free or low fat cottage cheese
Beans, nuts, seeds	1/4 cup beans 1/4 cup or 1 ounce nuts, seeds
Lean meat, fish, poultry, eggs count ounces of cooked meat, fish, poultry	3 ounces are about the size of a deck of cards or the palm of a woman's hand 1 egg = 1 oz, 2 egg whites = 1 oz
Fats, fatty sauces	1 tablespoon salad dressing 1 teaspoon butter, oil

Index

About the Author

Marla Heller is a Registered Dietitian, and holds a Master of Science in Human Nutrition and Dietetics from the University of Illinois at Chicago (UIC), where she is completing course work on a PhD in Behavior Sciences and Health Promotion. She owns Transitions Nutrition Consulting and provides individual nutrition counseling to hundreds of people every year. She has been an adjunct clinical instructor at UIC, Dominican University, National-Louis University, and the Cooking and Hospitality Institute of Chicago.

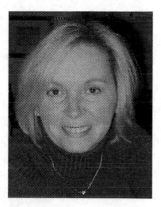

In addition to "The DASH Diet Action Plan," Marla wrote the 4-week menu plan for "Win the Weight Game" by Sarah, the Duchess of York. She has been a featured nutrition expert for the Chicago Tribune, Washington Post, and WGN-AM. She frequently presents seminars at corporations, schools, health clubs, and athletic facilities and is a spokesperson for the Greater Midwest Affiliate of the American Heart Association.

She is a Past-President of the Illinois Dietetic Association, and is a Past-President of the North Suburban Dietetic Association. She was recently awarded the prestigious Emerging Leader Award from the Illinois Dietetic Association.

Marla was diagnosed with high blood pressure in May of 2003. Since that time she has managed to keep her blood pressure in the normal range by following the DASH diet, losing 14 pounds, and exercising. Marla lives the program that is featured in her book, The DASH Diet Action Plan and seminars.

Marla lives with her husband, Richard in Northbrook, where she enjoys cooking, gardening, exercising, and writing.